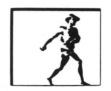

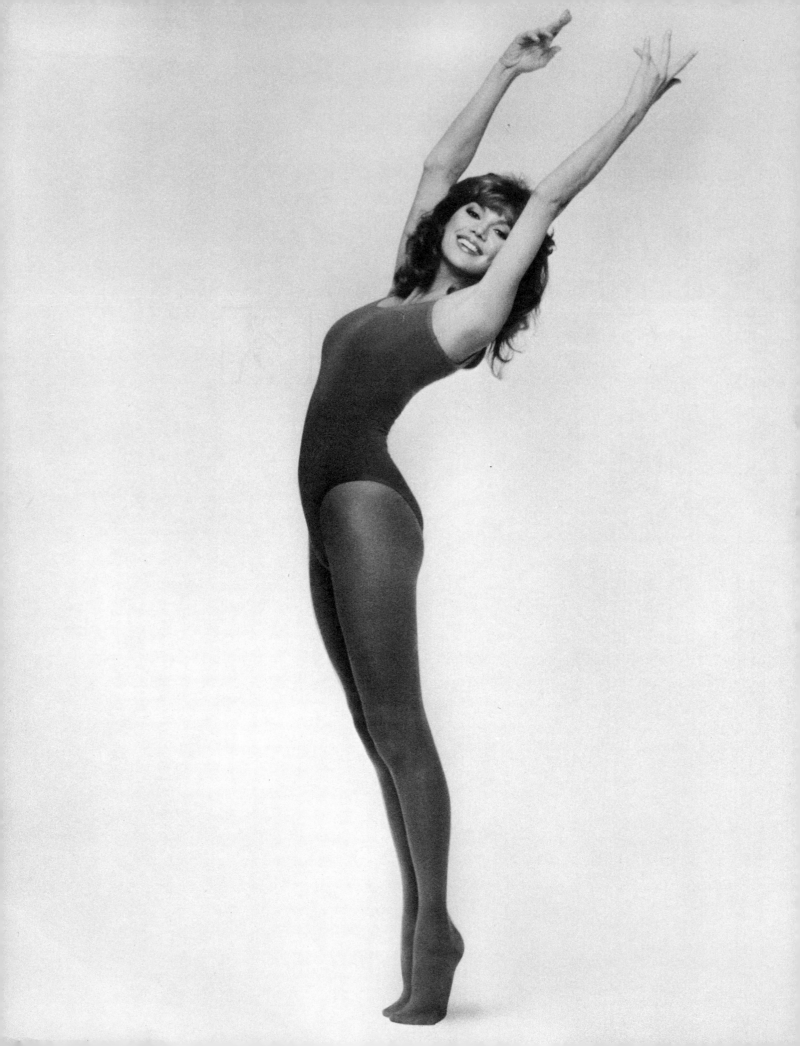

THE BODY PRINCIPAL

Victoria Principal

Photographs by HARRY LANGDON

SIMON AND SCHUSTER • NEW YORK

Copyright © 1983 by Pryce Hill Principal Productions, Inc.
All rights reserved
including the right of reproduction
in whole or in part in any form
Published by Simon and Schuster
A Division of Simon & Schuster, Inc.
Simon & Schuster Building
Rockefeller Center
1230 Avenue of the Americas
New York, New York 10020
SIMON AND SCHUSTER and colophon are registered trademarks of Simon & Schuster, Inc.
Designed by Eve Metz
Production directed by Jeanne Palmer
Manufactured in the United States of America

10   9   8   7   6   5   4

Library of Congress Cataloging in Publication Data
Principal, Victoria.
    The body principal.

    1.Reducing exercises.   2.Exercise for women.
3.Isometric exercise.   4.Reducing diets.   5.Principal,
Victoria.   6.Television personalities—United States—
Biography.   I.Title.
RA781.6.P74   1983   613.7'1   83-9436
ISBN 0-671-46684-4

All photographs by Harry Langdon, except page 123 © Norbert Jobst; page 19 © Scott Downie.
All photographs of exercise machines taken at Holiday Health Spa, Health and Tennis Corporation
of America. Hair by José Eber and Steve West; makeup by Marja Webster; styled by Suzie Biles.

Illustrations by Lamont A. O'Neal.

To my mother and father, without whom there would be no body Principal.

I love you.

ACKNOWLEDGMENTS

There are so many people I would like to thank for their help in making this book possible: Annie Gilbar, my very good friend, for her invaluable contribution; Sylvia Gold, for her unswerving belief in me; Jerry Edelstein, for believing anything is possible (and making it happen); Dan Green, for giving me a hard time . . . in the best way possible; Esther Newberg, who makes a great deal; Don Wildman, who has been a wonderful example and an inspiration to me; Leonard Katzman, my producer and friend, whose influence, support and encouragement touches everything I do; Wally Bregman, president of Playtex, who can do no wrong; Harry Langdon, who brings to every photograph the beauty that is in his own soul; José Eber, for his years of friendship (to me and my hair); Dr. Donald Schwartz, Dr. Paul Ward, Dr. Bruce Oppenheim, Dr. Sandra Aronberg, Marja Webster, Steve West, Angela Piervencenti, Angela Sabbaghi (Lucy), Suzie Biles, Alan Nierob, George Kirvay . . . and my Harry.

CONTENTS

Foreword by Donald Schwartz, M.D., 9

Chapter 1—The Early Principal   **11**

Chapter 2—The Body Principles   **20**
Body Resistive Exercises, 22
Convenience and Ease, 24
Organizing Your Own Program, 28
Completion of the Exercise Sets, 29
Pain and Injury, 30
Breathing, 31
Music, 32
Mirrors, 32
Shedding Your Clothes, 34
Moderation, 34
Exercise and Travel, 35

Chapter 3—The Exercise Sets   **36**
Warm-ups, 42
Set I—Buttocks and Pelvis, 56
Set II—Arms, Forearms, Shoulders, and Chest, 60
Set III—Calves and Ankles, 66
Set IV—Stomach (Lower Abdomen) and Thighs, 74
Set V—Upper Abdomen, 82
Set VI—Waist, 84
Set VII—Thighs, 90
Set VIII—Shoulders, 98
Set IX—Knees, 100
Set X—Hamstrings, 102
Set XI—Chest and Breasts, 104
Set XII—Breathing, 106
Warm-down, 108

Chapter 4—Sports in Your Life: The Options   **110**
Some Hints on Choosing a Sport, 112
Begin at the Beginning, 113
How Often, 113
Wearing a Bra, 114
Warm-ups, 115

The Choices: Swimming, 117
        Tennis and Racquetball, 119
        Skiing, 122
        Bicycling, 125
        Golf, 127
        Bowling, 129
        Running, 131
        Football, Baseball, Basketball and Volleyball, 134

Chapter 5—Exercise Machines: The Options   136

The Truth About Exercise Machines, 139
Hints for Exercising with Machines, 141
Knee Extension, 144
Shoulder Press, 146
Leg Curl, 148
Pull-down, 150
Leg Press, 152
Chest Press, 154
Rotary Torso Machine, 156
Push-down, 158
Hip-and-Back Machine, 160
Abdominal Machine, 162
Vertical Fly, 164
High Chair, 166

Chapter 6—The 30-Day Diet for Life   168

Sensible Is Best, 168
Moderation and Balance: The Secret to Nutrition, 171
Food Is Fuel, 171
Rules to Eat By, 173
Forbidden Foods, 173
Principles of The 30-Day Diet for Life, 176
Seven-Day Menu, 180
Food Chart, 183
It Works, 184

Chapter 7—A Life Style of Maintenance   185

Physical and Mental Harmony, 185
Sex and Exercise, 188
Exercising Forever, 191

Foreword

For centuries exercise has been recognized as necessary for a healthy body. In recent years common sense has often been abandoned in determining ways to exercise the body. Various fads, ranging from running excessively to extreme weight-training programs, and, more recently, aerobics, have led to injuries in millions of people.

The Body Principal Program is based on the principle of isometric contraction. This process involves tightening the muscle without actually moving the adjacent joint. This builds up a resistance and stress within the muscle and is a safe method of exercising and toning it. Individual muscles can be worked efficiently in a very controlled manner, and the degree of muscle development can be determined by the frequency and intensity of repetitions performed.

It has been my experience as an orthopedic surgeon, having observed and treated high school, collegiate and professional athletes for many years, that the importance of safe and controlled exercises, such as those in The Body Principal Program, cannot be overemphasized. Victoria's exercises can be performed safely and conveniently, at home or at work, with great effectiveness. They are presented in a manner that can be understood and practiced easily. They allow you to concentrate on specific body areas, reshaping and toning them comfortably with virtually no risk of injury.

The Body Principal Program introduces a well-conceived warm-up routine prior to the beginning of exercising. It is essential to warm up adequately before any exercise activity in order to prevent injury. A good warm-up is critical because when a muscle is cold it is not able to stand stress, thus causing the muscle to tear instead of stretch.

Women's participation in regular exercise programs has rapidly increased in popularity. Now is the ideal time for a program such as Victoria's because of its unique advantages for working women, for women with small children who have limited time, and for any women who are interested in a simple, effective, convenient and fun program of exercise. The Body Principal approach can successfully aid women in developing their own exercise format based on their individual needs.

Victoria's Body Principal is a commonsense method for safe, effective, healthy exercise on a regular basis.

—Donald Schwartz, M.D.
Orthopedic Surgery
Cedars-Sinai Medical Center
Los Angeles, California

CHAPTER 1

The Early Principal

Every day of my life, just as I eat, just as I sleep, just as I work, just as I love—I exercise.

I am a very busy woman. I have a full-time career, run my own home, do my own cooking, lead an active social life and regularly volunteer my services to my community. I am over thirty, and I am in *great shape!* This is no accident—my parents have given me many things, but a perfect body is not one of them. My body is in great shape because I have discovered that being in excellent condition—with muscles toned, skin tight, body trim and strong—is easier and much more fun than you may think. And the rewards are enormous.

Let's be honest. Many of us are not in as great shape as we were at sixteen. (And if you are still sixteen, go look in the mirror and memorize how you look; or better yet, take a snapshot, because no matter what you think now, it's not going to last forever!) Some of us are lazy, and all of us are, to one degree or another, very busy.

But being permanently older than sixteen and part-time lazy and full-time busy doesn't mean we have to be out of shape. It has always been my belief that a woman who complains that she is hungry when dieting or that her body hurts if she exercises is likely to be the same person who wears shoes that kill her feet. Fitness begins with a conscious decision to make it a top priority in your life. Remember: You can take off those shoes, but taking off those thighs takes a lot more doing.

Taking off those flabby thighs or unattractive extra pounds does not have to be difficult or time-consuming. You do not have to submit to daily, hour-long exercise classes, jogging sessions, bike rides, fasting ordeals or sore muscles. Exercise can be easy, affordable, fast, effective and fun. Over the years and out of necessity, I have developed for myself an exercise program that, when practiced in a special, relatively simple way, has become an unobtrusive routine in my life and has resulted in a toned, tight resculpted body that is in its best condition ever.

It wasn't always so. Up until a few years ago, I did not exercise. I played tennis, I swam, I hunted, and I worked, worked and worked some more. I guess I always figured that my body would stay as tight and as firm as it was when I was sixteen.

It didn't.

One Saturday morning a week before my twenty-ninth birthday, I was in my kitchen in jeans, making breakfast for my best friend, Annie. As I was beating the eggs, Annie walked in, looked at me strangely from behind, and with some nonchalance said, "What's that thing on your legs?" I looked around, looked again, and then realized that the thing she was talking about was my bottom.

I was shocked. As recently as I had been able to remember, my reasonably attractive bottom had been in its proper place. But as I now looked where Annie was pointing, I realized that without my even noticing it, my bottom had fallen. "How could this have happened to my body without my being aware of it?" I thought to myself. After all, my body was with me at all times. How could I have been so blind? Leaving Annie with the unscrambled eggs, I ran upstairs to my bedroom, took off my shirt and jeans, and stood in front of my mirror naked. Sure enough, there it was—someone else's body, a body that was definitely in need of some remodeling.

I sat down on the bed. "This is serious," I thought. When was the last time I exercised? I couldn't remember. All right—when was the first time I exercised? For some reason, that one was easier.

I was thirteen, sitting on a towel by the swimming pool at a club near my house in Georgia, my girlfriend Julie by my side. At this club, the rule was that if you didn't have a towel (or a mat), you couldn't sit by the pool. Suddenly a rather large boy came by and yanked my towel away. I was furious. But he was bigger—it was obvious that I was either going to stand in the sun all day or go home. But Julie jumped up, picked up this big kid and threw him into the pool. Was I impressed! I never knew she was that strong. As the now-humiliated young man slithered away in amazement, Julie proceeded to explain that since she was on the swimming team, she worked out with weights to strengthen her arm muscles. Naturally, I immediately ran out to buy two small hand weights, and for years, I used them every now and then to do the simple lifts and press exercises that Julie had taught me. That was the extent of my exercise program.

My mother, Ree, exercised. I remember I would come home from school and there she would be, down on the floor in the living room, doing her exercises to music. I never could understand why she was down there so much of the time, since I had always assumed that she came by her impressive body naturally, and that mine would also stay firm and tight, just as it was.

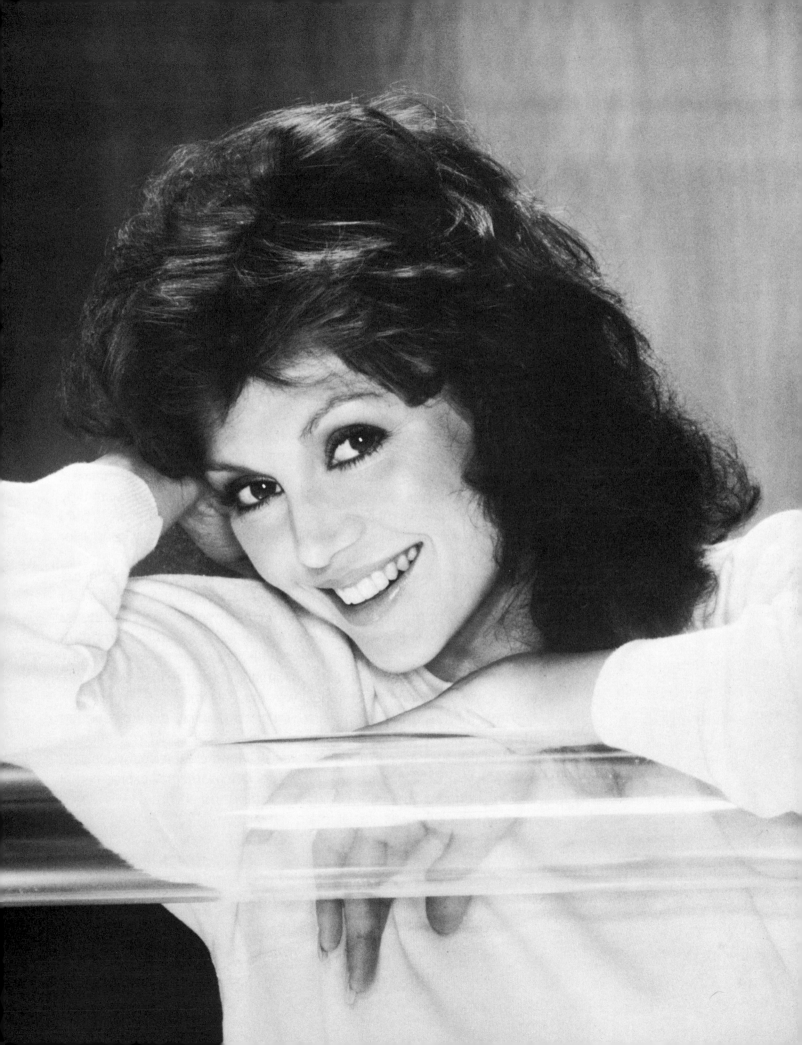

A few years went by. I took up sports of all sorts—I swam, played basketball, volleyball and tennis. Then, when I was eighteen, I gained some weight. When the modeling agency I was working with asked me to lose it—and fast—I assumed that it would go away . . . and eventually it did. Meanwhile, I still kept active. I would go dancing Friday night until there was no place open. On Saturday I would go to the Everglades and hunt until noon, then rush home, shower, and meet my friends at the beach, where I would water-ski for six hours at a stretch. When the sun went down, off I would go to the Jockey Club until it closed. Then came Sunday, and I would swim and play touch football, come home to wash and wax my car, then go to work on Monday. Yet I didn't exercise—that is, I did no specific work for the different parts of my body.

The years passed. Then I had an accident. It was 1977. I was on vacation in Hawaii, playing football, when somebody threw a rolling block and I didn't get out of the way in time. I hurt my right knee and had to be flown back to Los Angeles immediately. The pain was awful! I went to two orthopedic surgeons and both said I had "slipped" a knee-cap out of joint, which resulted in a weakened quadriceps muscle (that's the one on the front of the thigh) and that I would have to have surgery. I am no fan of surgery unless there is absolutely no other alternative. I am also not a fan of scars—I was petrified that I would end up with ugly knees for life! I knew that surgery was a real quick way to get well, but I also felt that it would probably limit my activities (especially sports) for the rest of my life.

I then went to see Dr. Donald Schwartz, another orthopedic surgeon, who felt that surgery was not necessary. He suggested that I wear a cast (from the top of my thigh to my ankle) for two weeks, stay on crutches for another two weeks, and then limit my activities for up to six months, during which time I had to see a physical therapist for an exercise program. Well, the first two I could handle—but limiting my active life (I was about to do a movie, among other things) was unbearable.

So we made a deal. Dr. Schwartz, understanding my determination to try to get better fast and my financial situation (I could not afford a physical therapist for six months), agreed to let me exercise myself back to health. He gave me a stack of papers with "isometric" exercises that would strengthen my injured muscles without hurting me. He warned me that exercising was crucial to a good recovery.

And six weeks later—I walked. I limped a little, but I walked. In just a few weeks (rather than a few months), by exercising my muscles, I recovered. At the end of three months I could actually put on a low pair of heels; although it was a year before I could wear high-heeled shoes, and well over a year before I could play sports again. With the resistive exercises, I had helped myself get well. But then I stopped exercising. I suppose I felt that since I was no longer injured, I no longer needed to exercise.

Several years passed. I stayed thin (105 to 110 pounds) even as I got older. By the time I was twenty-eight, I was starring in "Dallas" and working constantly. My days began at 5:30 A.M. and often ended at 7 at night. I worked five or six days a week, twelve months a year. I was busier than I had ever been. But I felt fine, looked pretty good, and except for some softening of my arm muscles (no time for tennis anymore) and some wrinkles on my thighs, I thought I was in good physical shape.

Then came the "Battle of the Network Stars." That was a show that pitted different stars from competing television networks in various difficult sporting events, with cash prizes to the winners. I was invited to be a contestant on the show, and I accepted without any reservations. Because I had always participated in so many sports, I had confidence in my strength and my ability to compete. I was certain that besides having a wonderful time, I could probably win in at least a few events, and return home with pride intact (and some cash in hand). So I accepted, and while we were filming in Dallas, I decided to get in shape.

One morning I woke up long before my 7 A.M. call and went for a run. I ran about fifteen yards and collapsed. I couldn't believe it! Fifteen yards! Me—the skinny lady with the stamina and the energy and the strength—I couldn't run a block! I was devastated. I stumbled back to my room in tears and decided to call NBC to cancel my appearance on the show. ("Hi there, this is Victoria Principal. I am sorry but I can't do the Battle of the Network Stars. You see, I'm much older than I thought!")

Then I remembered I could use the money. So I decided to train. I immediately joined the President's Health Club in Dallas and started going religiously, hoping to get my body in shape. When we returned to Los Angeles, I began swimming at UCLA every morning. By the time the show was taped, I competed—and I won.

I was exhilarated and very proud of myself, particularly because I had forgotten how much fun it was to push my body and to have it prove equal to the task. As a kid, you run around all day, constantly straining your body without a second thought. But as you get older, it's not so easy. After that first show, I became motivated. I loved winning, and I loved the shape my body was in, the renewed strength it had. But I still couldn't find the time to go to exercise classes. Thus, every time I would be invited to compete on "Battle of the Network Stars" I would work out before the show, do well, and finally collapse.

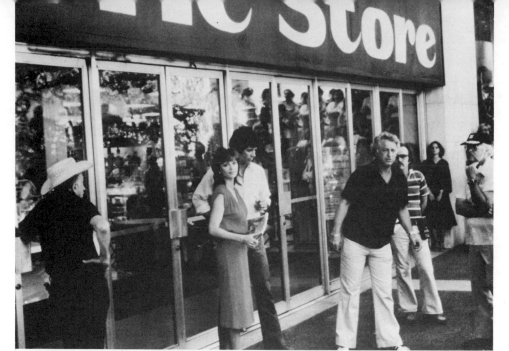

On location
in Dallas with my
costar Patrick Duffy

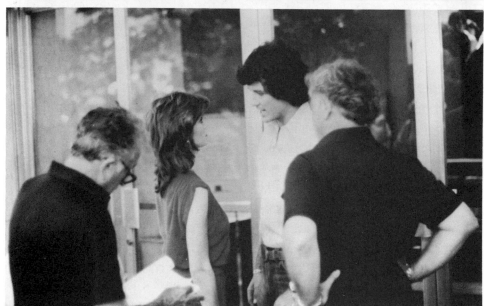

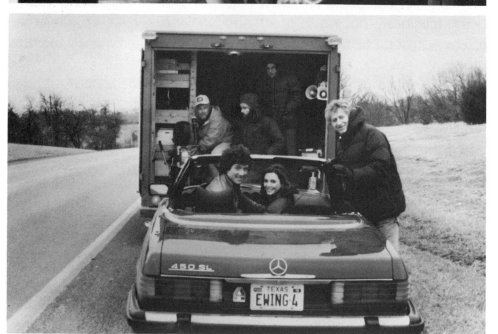

The first day, the first
shot, of a miniseries that
became "Dallas"

After the last show, I promised myself I'd stay in good shape. But as usual, work interrupted my plans. "Dallas" became a hit, and my schedule was overloaded. There was the show, and there were public appearances, interviews, commercials, movies. In addition I ran my house, and there was no time, I thought, to watch out for my body. I certainly did not have time for an elaborate daily routine of exercises I didn't care about and didn't think I needed, and I didn't want to take the chance of getting hurt and missing work. So I did no exercise at all.

Then Annie's comment about my bottom jolted me into realizing I needed to do something. If I wanted a better body, I had to figure out a way to stay in shape that would work for me. I wanted to reshape my body, and I had to do it in a way that would fit my busy schedule; it had to be convenient, flexible and fun. If this was at all possible, I was going to find a way.

I began by approaching everyone I knew for advice. I asked doctors, chiropractors, friends, actors, dancers, body builders, exercise instructors: What did they do to keep their bodies in shape? I went from gym to gym, from exercise class to dance class to aerobics class—to discover the different methods people used. Finally I realized that something I had believed for a long time (proven to me when I hurt my knee) was true: Only I really know how my body works, how it responds to exercise; that, indeed, each of us is the best judge of how our muscles work. I found that I knew what was best for me, that I could feel what parts of my body needed tightening and toning and how far I could go in my body work.

The first exercise I found was one dancers use to tighten their thighs and keep their buttocks firm and high. I tried it and found it worked for me. By experimenting, I found that this same exercise, done in other positions, contracted and toned other muscles. I saw a difference in my own muscle tone almost immediately—and I was in heaven! Next was my fallen bottom. I found that this is a common occurrence especially among women; that it happens as a woman's body matures, because, if there is no counterforce to stop it, a muscle will naturally fall over time. But I also found that this "natural falling" is easily stopped and/or reversed by simple resistive exercises that use your own force to tone and tighten these muscles. I found that I could actually firm and lift my own fallen bottom. I could, and I did.

And that was the beginning. Slowly, carefully, with determination and excitement, I collected more and more exercises for each part of the body, exercises that I can do anywhere, that require no equipment, that take little time, that are fun to do—and that work!

Today I exercise every day—happily, easily, enthusiastically—and the results are better than I would ever have dreamed possible. I am leaner and look taller. Now when I move, my body moves with me. I also look better in clothes; you yourself know the difference between clothes that contain, or hide, your body (like those skintight jeans that really work as a girdle) and skin that contains your body (when everything is just the way it should be and there's nothing to hide). My body is in better shape than it was when I was sixteen—it is firmer, shapelier and stronger.

And it's not just my imagination. Everywhere I go, people ask me how I keep in shape. On the "Dallas" set, members of the cast notice me doing exercises between takes, and they start doing them, too. A saleswoman in a department store told me about her "problem thighs." I showed her the thigh exercises she could do while at work—and when I returned just a couple of weeks later, she was busy toning her body and the results already showed. I met a manicurist who complained that her buttocks had fallen after years of sitting on the job. Three weeks and many buttocks exercises later, her bottom was on its way to renewed firmness (accomplished, let me remind you, while she was at work). One of the makeup artists I work with saw me doing my unobtrusive exercises as she applied my makeup, started doing them while she worked—and became a firmer, shapelier devotee. Sometimes on commercial shoots, I end up giving exercise classes in my trailer—simply by showing people how they can do resistive exercises for their bodies at home.

My exercises also help me to release the tension and stress that build up in the body daily. Exercising (especially when you enjoy it) is the best way I know for relaxing at the end of the day. My program gives me renewed energy that makes me a more productive and happier person. I have found that I now have excellent control over my muscles, that I have more strength, a more satisfying sex life and a better self-image. I look better, I *am* better.

I don't encourage you to look like me; but I do encourage you to take better care of yourself. For me—when my mind is in tune with my body (and you know how it feels when that happens), when I have physical and mental harmony (and one *does* depend on the other), that is when I look my best. Not just for the camera, but for myself.

Following the exercise principles that I have formulated has changed my life. I hope that you, too, can use these body principles to change yours.

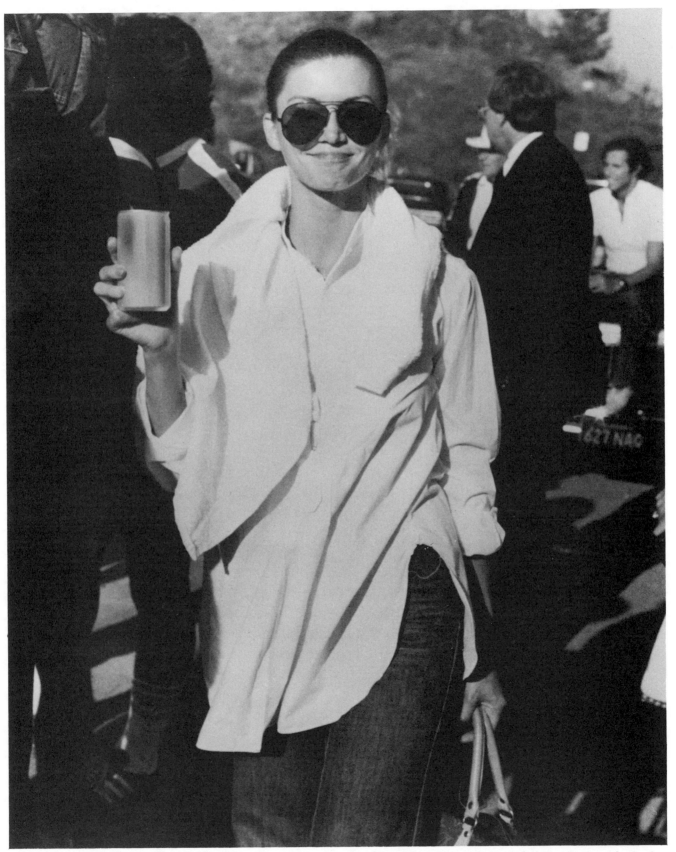

The first "Battle of the Network Stars"—the joy of winning

CHAPTER 2
The Body Principles

The body principles are really life principles, basic guidelines that make exercising a habitual, comfortable, effective and enjoyable part of our lives. The principles are based on common sense; they advocate only the natural, sane and safe ways to tone, tighten and resculpt your body. They are based on the assumption that you know your body best; that resculpting your body, making it look the way you want it to look, is within your control; that you can choose those parts of your body you want to change; that you will know how far you can go, how much your muscles can and should do; that you can put together an exercise program individually designed for your life style, your schedule and your body.

These principles recognize that our lives are busy; thus, they advocate and illustrate an exercise program that is flexible—one that you can do virtually anywhere, that you can alter when it is necessary, and that you will never outgrow (you can do these exercises forever—the better you get at them, the more you do of them). It is an exercise routine that bends to accommodate your schedule and requirements—you don't change your routine for the exercises. It is founded on my belief that, given the choice, you would rather be fit and toned, and as beautiful as you can be—easily, comfortably, naturally and painlessly.

It may sound too good to be true: exercises that are natural to the body, easy to do and safe, take little time and can be done anywhere—and work! Actually resistive exercises have been around for a long time, perhaps because they are so safe and so effective. What makes my program different and universally applicable is that I have chosen resistive exercises for each part of the body and have formulated a program that is flexible; you can put your own exercise routine together to reshape and resculpt your individual body.

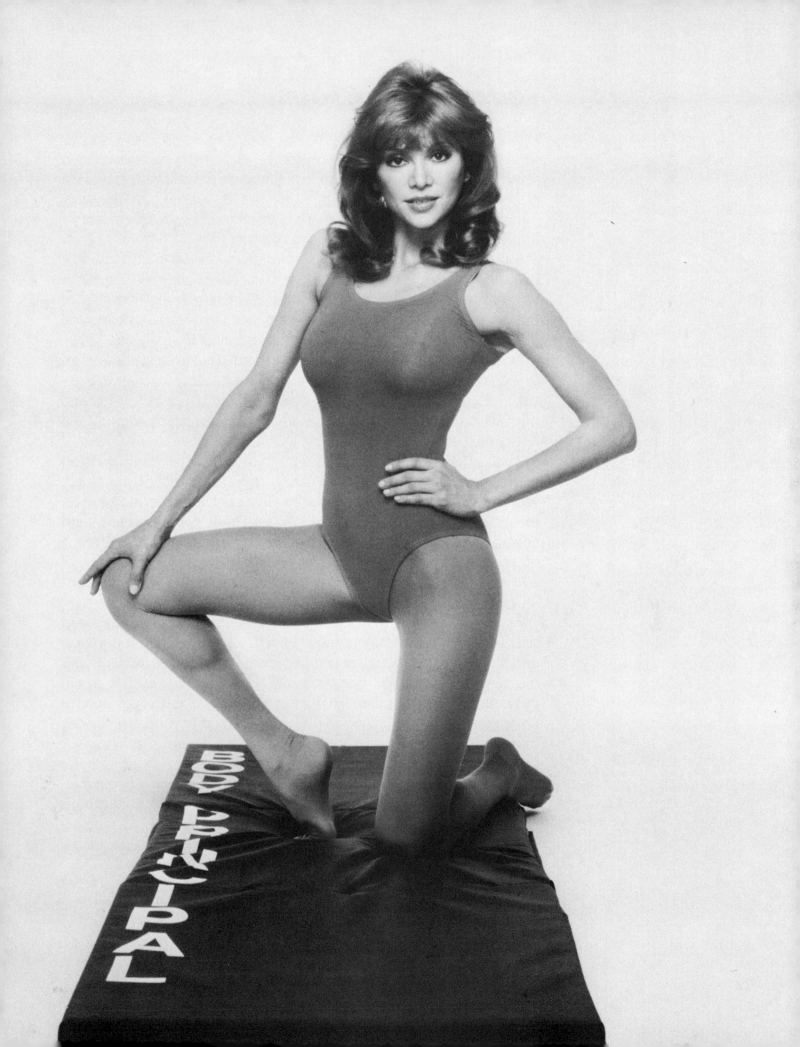

BODY RESISTIVE EXERCISES

First let me explain what body resistive exercises—also called isometrics—are. Isometrics are based on the belief that the contraction and stretching of muscles are important, and that resistance of forces against muscles results in toned and firmer muscles. By working an individual muscle in a static position—slowly and with attention only to that muscle—it will be strengthened and tightened naturally.

Muscles waste away without use. Not to use a muscle is to lose it. If you ever visit an injured friend in the hospital (especially one who is in a cast), you will find that his or her muscles are atrophying from lack of use. Your muscles waste away and your bones can become osteoporotic (they lose calcium and become brittle) as a result of inactivity.

Not great news. That is why both injured patients and those with various bone diseases are encouraged to do isometric, or resistive, exercises. These exercises strengthen dormant muscle tissues on isolated muscles naturally—without undue strain or movement throughout the rest of the body.

Try this. Take one hand and place it against your other hand, pressing them together. This is resistance. As you are pressing, feel the muscles in your upper arms contracting. By doing this continuous resistive movement, you are getting *total resistance*—that muscle is contracting (and tightening) the entire time you are pressing your hands against each other. With this total resistance, you are making the most efficient use of your energy—you are expending maximum energy and getting maximum results.

As you contract the muscle, the fibers move together and increase in size; you don't develop more muscle fibers, just larger ones. It is important to understand the difference between exercises that resculpt your muscles and those that create larger, often bulging muscles. The aim in this exercise program is to redefine muscles, to tone them, and to reduce or enlarge them as you choose. (If you wish to go beyond toning your muscles to properly enlarge them using weights and/or machines, see Chapter 5.)

I don't want eighteen-inch biceps or calves that resemble watermelons. But I do want tight muscle tone. By repeating my contractions (without adding any extra weights) slowly and continuously, I am developing muscles that have a tighter, stronger linear definition rather than a bigger bulge. I am actually working with my body, not against it.

Cellulite, or fatty deposits, is those flabby, lumpy, rippling rolls that settle most often on the hips, thighs and legs. Although there has been some

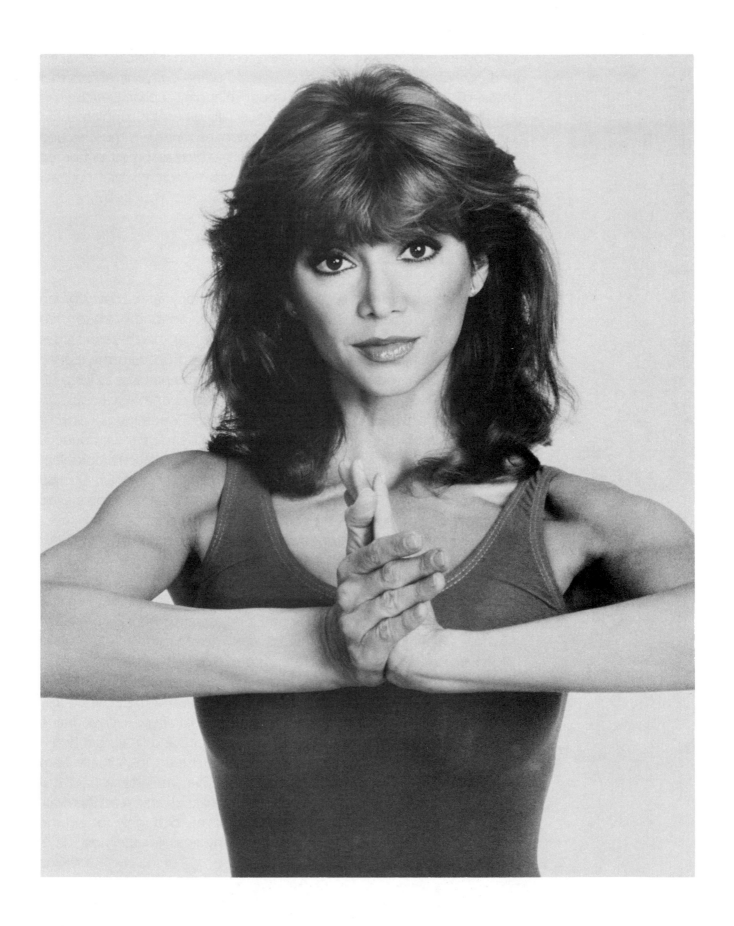

controversy over the years about the existence of what we call "cellulite," and conflicting views about how to get rid of it—everyone agrees that these rolls of fat don't simply wave goodbye and disappear. Exercise can help the body eliminate this extra fat, especially when it is supplemented by occasional local massage. Resistive exercises tone your muscles and in the process cause your small fatty deposits to be reabsorbed, or burned up, by turning them into energy. Thus, resistive exercises that contract and tighten your muscles can result in redefinition of your body.

CONVENIENCE AND EASE

My exercise routines can be done by anyone at any time. Busy women and working women, who take pride in their bodies and want to keep in shape or who want to reshape their bodies, can do these exercises any time and almost anywhere. It is easy to keep up with my regime because there are no classes to go to, so there is no pressure to keep up with others (who has not tried to overcompensate for awkwardness by trying too hard?); there are no instructors who know nothing about your body, urging you to try still harder; you won't have to deal with general exercises that are not specifically directed at your particular problem areas; and the possibility of injury is greatly minimized. As Dr. Donald Schwartz explains: "These exercises are particularly safe for people who may have clinical problems they don't know about, such as weak knees or a weak lower back." And best of all—there is no more planning your day around a class that is arranged according to someone else's schedule.

The principle here is convenience—to make it easy to exercise. Convenience was an important reason for my formulating this exercise program. My schedule, like yours, is full. I spend long, grueling hours on my feet. My days start at 5:30 in the morning, when I get up to drive to the set at MGM studios. (Believe me, there are no exercise classes being held at that hour!) After having my makeup and hair done, I start work. At 1 P.M. I return to my dressing room for an hour lunch and some exercise (my makeup and hair remain intact—just as yours would after exercises during your lunch hour at your office). I return to work at 2 and finally get home at approximately 7 P.M. If I feel like it, I then exercise again. Actually, I am a great fan of exercising in the evening. It revives me after a hard day and prepares me for the night ahead. Then I make dinner, read the mail, return phone calls and eventually collapse on my bed (only to find the script waiting for me so I can memorize my lines for the next day's shooting).

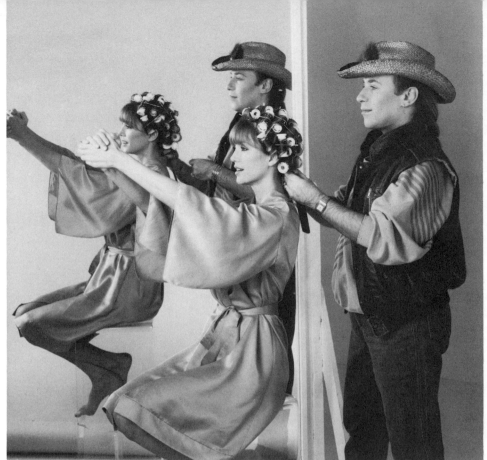

Here I am exercising
while José Eber
does my hair.

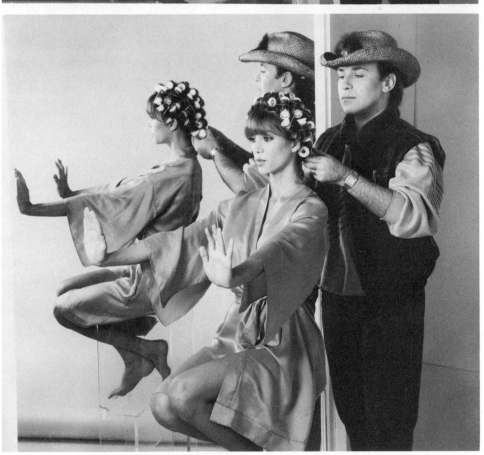

I also exercise while
Marja Webster
makes me up.

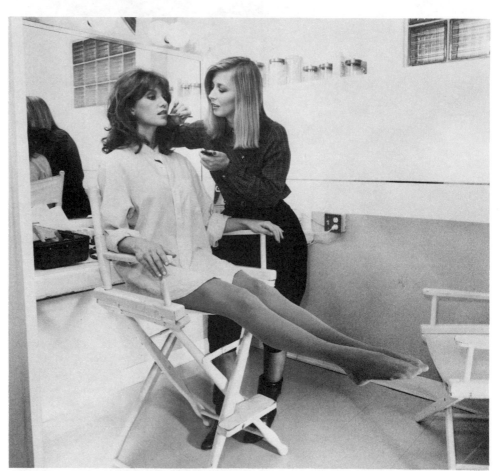

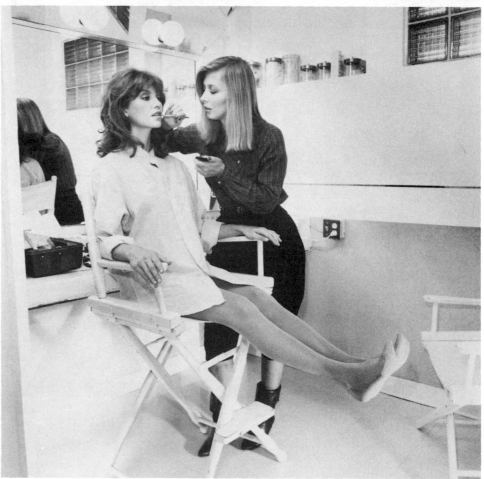

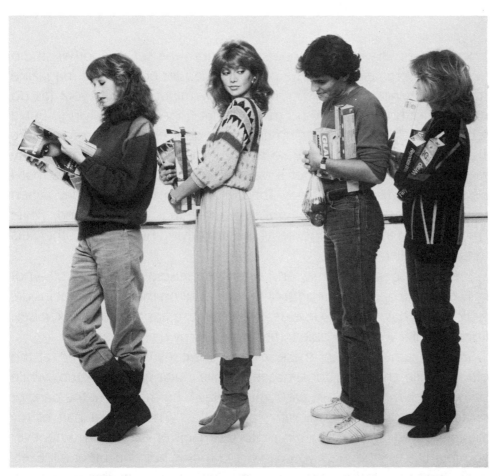

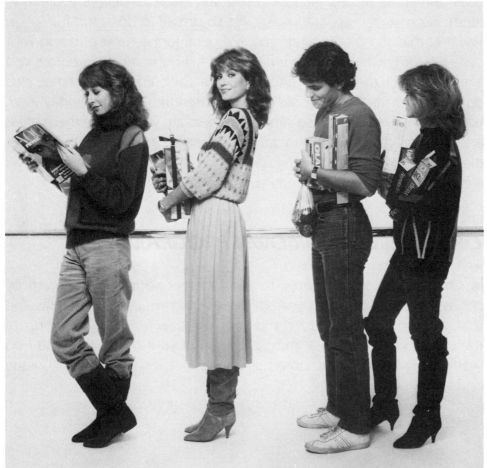

You can exercise, just like me,
while standing in line
at the grocery store.

Sometimes I have to continue straight from the set to another studio to shoot a commercial or to be photographed for print ads or magazine stories. I am not complaining. I love every minute of my work (as do many other busy women, no matter what they do for a living). But a schedule such as this leaves no time for organized exercise of any sort. That's why my programs are so terrific! I manage to set aside twenty minutes in the morning after I wake up for a complete routine that I designed for my problem areas. Then, in addition, during the day, when I have the time (for example, while my makeup is being applied, while I'm talking on the telephone, or while I am driving home), I do other sets that I have selected.

I really do believe that when I wasn't exercising, it took its toll—not only on the shape and strength of my body but on the stress I kept inside, which now has a healthy release. If it weren't so easy to do my exercises, I don't think I would be able to fit them into my daily schedule.

You too can do any of these resistive exercises in your home, at the office, while shopping for groceries, while putting on makeup, while sitting at the movies, while vacuuming, watching the kids at the park, or driving your car—the possibilities are endless. The hardest part of my routine is beginning it—getting into the habit of exercising whenever you feel like it, whenever you can—and that is not difficult at all. Exercises don't have to be torture, and you don't have to devote your life to them. Because my sets of exercises are so simple to do—and fun—you will find that, in no time at all, you will get into the habit of doing your own full routine at the same time each day (in the morning before you eat breakfast, in the evening after work or at the office at lunchtime), plus doing other particular exercises you've chosen throughout the day. And, because the exercises are so simple, chances are you will do them often and thus see the results on your body quickly. And remember: Rather than altering your busy schedule or life style, these resistive exercises will easily fit into your everyday routine.

ORGANIZING YOUR OWN PROGRAM

In Chapter 3, I describe how to put together your own program by choosing sets of exercises geared to reshaping your problem areas and that you will have time to do in your full day. (A set is made up of exercises for one particular muscle or area of your body.) But here I do want to explain why the individual nature of this program is so unique and important.

These exercises are divided into sets that are tailored to specific muscles or muscle groups for certain parts of your body (that is, stomach muscles, thighs, upper arms, calves, buttocks, shoulders, abdomen, waist, knees, hamstrings, chest). By choosing a set to resculpt a specific part of your body, say the calves, you know exactly what you are doing and exactly which muscles you are working on. By pinpointing those parts of your body that are your problem areas and selecting the sets of exercises specifically designed to tone those areas, you are formulating your own program that will reshape your body the way you want.

These exercises are safe and sane—it is hard to hurt yourself. All you have to do is do the exercises, and your body will be reshaped and toned.

It is my belief that you are the best judge of your body. You know what you like about it and what you don't like. You are aware of your muscles—how they work, how they tighten and how they stretch—and you are able to determine the force and pressure of your muscles as no exercise teacher in a class ever can. After doing these exercises for a while, you will also be an expert at more subtle pressure changes in your muscle tone as your body gets firmer. These are *commonsense* exercises—there is nothing difficult, dangerous or unnatural about them. You don't *need* a checkup from your doctor, but a regular checkup is a good idea. These simple, safe exercises work your muscles naturally and sensibly.

You know yourself best, so take charge of your life and forge ahead. For a more detailed explanation of how to formulate your own resistive exercise routine, see the introduction in Chapter 3: "The Exercise Sets."

COMPLETION OF THE EXERCISE SETS

It is important to maintain momentum once you start a set of exercises. Because this program is so flexible, it is possible not only to do your entire routine of sets but also to isolate one muscle and do the exercise for toning it at any time (as long as you always remember to warm up first). The important principle is to *finish* each set you start. Don't stop in the middle of a set—not even if the phone rings (they'll call back)—or for any reason other than an emergency (picking up a crying child or stopping at a red light counts as an emergency). If you are doing your sets in the office, close the door and insist on not being interrupted. If you don't have a private office, a lounge or ladies' room will do.

Let me repeat: Once you start your exercise sets, try to keep the momentum going so your contractions and stretches are completed each and every time you start them. If you must stop for a moment or stop completely for the day, do so after you have finished the set. If you get tired, just do them more slowly—but finish the set. You will find that finishing an exercise is helpful for developing discipline and for getting results in your toning program.

PAIN AND INJURY

"Safe and sane" is my motto. It is very difficult to get hurt doing these resistive exercises because you are performing a natural movement. Contracting and stretching your muscles is natural; they are related movements. For example, when you contract the front thigh muscles, the hamstrings, the tendons attached to the muscles in back of your thighs, stretch naturally and automatically. You are not adding additional weights, and you don't jerk the muscles or move quickly and randomly. With these exercises, you do only as much as you can, and you are the best judge of how much you can and should do. You can best determine how much force you can exert because you are aware of your body's condition. Contracting (toning) the muscle slowly, continuously and repetitively is a natural movement; there is nothing artificial about it. After a while your muscles get used to this movement; you feel as if they expect it—and that means they are getting toned.

I've spoken about the use of resistive exercises in hospitals, specifically because you can't get hurt by doing them. It should also be noted that when doing these exercises you will rarely feel sore the next day. This requires a bit of explaining. According to Dr. Bruce Oppenheim, a well-known chiropractor (he also happens to be mine), you might consider this analogy: When your car burns gas, the result is that it moves. Another result is that carbon monoxide, a poisonous gas is released. When you contract a muscle too much, which happens in many classes where you do ordinary exercises, you burn up the sugar and oxygen in that muscle. The byproduct of an extensive muscle contraction is lactic acid, and it is this accumulation of acid that causes sore muscles. Dr. Donald Schwartz explains: "When you exercise in aerobics or other conventional exercise techniques, you take in enough oxygen to supply adequate energy for what you are doing. As you continue to exercise rapidly, you need energy at a faster rate than you can produce it. At such a point you are producing energy without oxygen—you are in *oxygen debt*. This oxygen debt results in a buildup of lactic acid, which irritates the muscle and makes it hurt. There is yet another kind of sore muscle and that is when you strain it by doing exercise beyond its capabilities. This happens often in exercise classes, and can result in injuries to those muscles."

This causes a vicious cycle—you exercise too hard, build up a certain amount of lactic acid, go into oxygen debt, and end up with sore muscles. But with The Body Principal Program resistive exercises, you don't overuse the muscles and never build up too much lactic acid. Thus you never go into oxygen debt, and you don't stress the muscles to the point of injury. The contracting action in resistive exercises is natural—it won't hurt your muscles. These somewhat passive exercises do not strain you.

To say that it is difficult to hurt yourself with resistive exercises is one thing; to say that there is never any pain is another. And, although I can safely say that there is no pain with resistive exercises, there is sometimes a pulling sensation that is beneficial. Here's why: The pain of injury is an obvious one—we know when we have been hurt. If you have ever broken an arm or torn a ligament or even sprained an ankle, you recognize the pain of injury.

Some pain, however, is beneficial, and that is the kind of pain that tells you your muscles are working. A pulling sensation or a contraction is something you *feel*. (If you think you're contracting, but you feel nothing, think again. You are probably not working that muscle at all.) With resistive exercises, you will not feel the pain of pushing yourself too hard; what you *will* feel is the sensation of your muscles working, and that's "good" pain.

One more thing: If you feel tired after doing a set of exercises, and you feel a pulling sensation (a "good" pain), flex your muscles or pull your knees to your chest. Walk around the room flexing your feet. These simple movements should relieve any uncomfortable feeling in your muscles. But rest assured that one of the best things about these exercises is that they are easy and painless.

BREATHING

Breathing is something we take for granted. It is reflexive and involuntary—your body will breathe whether or not you think about it. But during exercising, we can often forget to breathe properly. What often happens is that when you contract a muscle, you hold your breath. When you hold a contraction for a count of 10, you may tend to hold your breath for a count of 10, too. That's a bad idea. Try to think about breathing—to make it a conscious action.

I believe in breathing noisily—it shows that you are working hard and that you are taking in-and-out breaths. Purposefully inhale and exhale audibly. Let the air whistle through your pursed lips. Don't hold back the noise, even though it may sound funny in the beginning; you may also end up holding back your breath. Not all the exercises require these audible sounds, but all require you to breathe.

These sounds don't mean that the exercises are difficult—they aren't. Most of them require simple contractions and releases, and almost no movement. But if you make a conscious effort to breathe, you'll be filling your lungs with air and your blood with oxygen, and that is good for your body.

MUSIC

Turn it on! Whenever you exercise, if it is at all possible (and if you respond to music), turn it on. The rhythmic beat of the music can help keep the movement of the exercise going, urge you on to finish the set, and keep the routine from becoming boring. I prefer music that makes my blood speed up. Then I'm ahead of the game; my circulation is already on the go! I love music that fills me with energy and makes me feel like moving. If you prefer Bach, that's fine. Choose the music you enjoy—it will make your exercise time more pleasant and more fun.

MIRRORS

Now I believe as much as the next person that pushing someone into exercising—even if it's yourself—is rather fruitless. You have to want to change your appearance; you have to want to resculpt your body, to change your habits so that you look and feel terrific. This is not always easy. Some of us need a little help, at least at first—the final push that makes us say, "I want to begin—now!" Want to know how I do it? Whenever I sense that I am avoiding exercising (when I phone friends I haven't seen in twenty years, balance a checkbook for the fourth time and go downstairs to the kitchen just to make sure it is still there), I make myself stand naked in front of the full-length mirror in my bathroom (I keep it there so that even when I don't particularly want to see myself, I can't avoid it).

Let's face it: That mirror never lies. It's all there—every extra ounce of fat, every tired, sagging muscle. After staring at the body in front of me, I turn full circle so that I can really see the things that aren't the way I would like them to be. And that's about all the incentive I need.

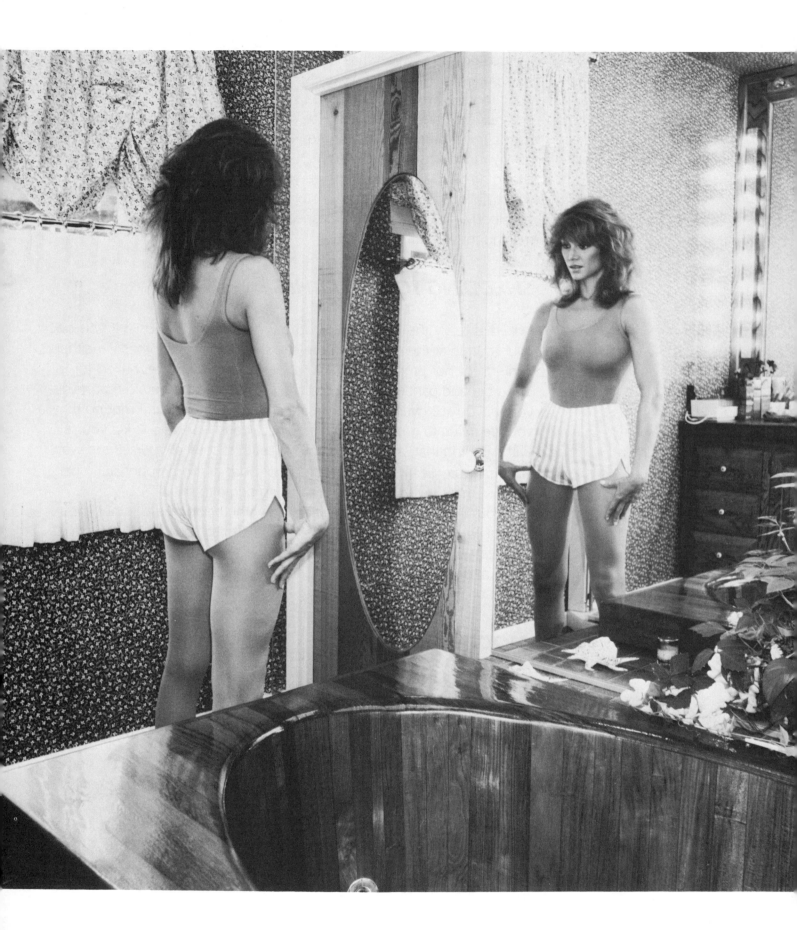

Also, looking at yourself as your body is being resculpted will reinforce your determination to keep exercising. Seeing the results will make you want to keep on going.

When you are exercising, try to do some of the sets in front of the mirror. It is a great way to learn to watch what your muscles are doing, how your body is moving, what is happening to those parts that you are changing. It is a revelation to see yourself in action—especially if you aren't hiding behind leotards or stockings or slacks. Get used to seeing your body—be proud of it! Be especially proud of the changes you are making for yourself.

SHEDDING YOUR CLOTHES

Naked is really the best way to do my exercises. Obviously, if you do your routine at the office or in the car, shedding your clothes is neither convenient nor proper. But if you are exercising at home, naked (or in just a bra and panties) is best. You can't hide behind a leotard that holds you in; you see every muscle, each inch of skin, every extra mound that you are trying to tone. You can see what needs work. Don't kid yourself with clothing that falsely holds you in. Learn to look at yourself the way you really are. Learn to be proud of your body—and prouder still when you see that the results of your exercising begin to show.

If you are exercising at the office, close the door, take off your shoes and, if you can, your panty hose (they restrict your movement; and besides, you'll make them baggy). The object here is to see your muscles work and to watch your skin tone up—not to watch the stretching action of Christian Dior.

MODERATION

Don't overdo it, but don't skimp either. I don't believe in overindulgence in anything (except maybe sex, if you are old enough). Moderation is best. I believe in a life of rewards, not denials. Any motion, especially exercising, is progress. It releases stress, it improves your self-image, it makes it hard to stagnate. Moreover, trying to overdo it in exercising is only going to tire you out. It is hard to hurt yourself with these exercises, but you can exhaust yourself.

So enjoy your life, and your exercising, by taking it easy. Results will come quickly, I assure you. There's no need to overdo, to rush, to do too much. It's a good lesson to learn and to apply to all parts of our lives. Take it easy and enjoy!

EXERCISE AND TRAVEL

For those of us who travel, be it by car, train or airplane, these sets of exercises are perfect. Resistive exercises have so little obvious movement that it is easy to do them anywhere. They are especially beneficial when you are stuck on an airplane for a long time. As you probably know, sitting in one position for hours is not good for your muscles or circulation. If you take the time to do some resistive sets while in this position, you will not only feel better during your trip, but you will also tone your body at the same time.

In Chapter 3, you will find that under each set of exercises I have listed the places where you can do that set or each of the exercises in it. Take note of which are convenient and proper to do in your car or on an airplane, so when you find yourself in these places, you will be prepared to use that valuable time to exercise easily and beneficially.

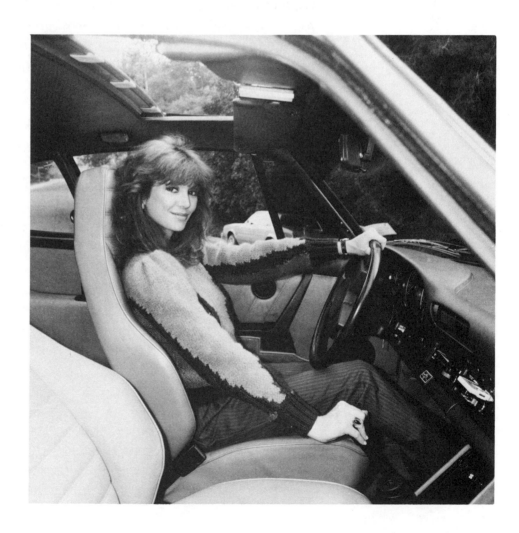

CHAPTER 3

The Exercise Sets

There are several decisions you need to make before you can put together your own individual exercise routine. First and foremost is deciding and listing which parts of your body you want to strengthen, tighten, tone and resculpt. Next you must determine how much time you can set aside in your day to do an exercise routine. Be honest—don't say thirty minutes when you know you'll never do more than fifteen or twenty minutes at one time. The wonderful thing about putting together this kind of exercise regime is that you don't have to limit yourself to the twenty minutes you may have in the morning before you eat your breakfast and have to be on your way. With this program you can put aside a certain time for your morning routine and still do other exercises at other times (and in various places) in the day.

Now that you know your time limit—let's say it's twenty minutes—and you have a list of the parts of the body you want to "reform," you are ready to put together your individual routine. The chart of The Body Principal Program lists all the exercises, the approximate time it takes to do them, and where they can be done. This is the total program that takes about twenty minutes.

A word here about time. Don't take my time calculations as law. If it takes you more (or less) time to do a specific exercise or a whole set—that's fine. My program may call for you to do the calf exercise on the stairs in one minute, but if it takes you a minute and a half or two minutes, don't force yourself to do it in one minute. Do the exercise in the minute and a half and figure that time into your entire program. Don't be intimidated by the time that is listed. You should know that the entire program *can* be done in twenty to thirty minutes. But what's more important is that you do the exercises at a speed that is comfortable for you without stress or strain.

Choosing your own combination of exercises to make up your routine (should the program as listed be too much for you) is a lot of fun. Suppose you want to concentrate on resculpting and reconditioning your buttocks and calves and tightening your thighs but have no interest

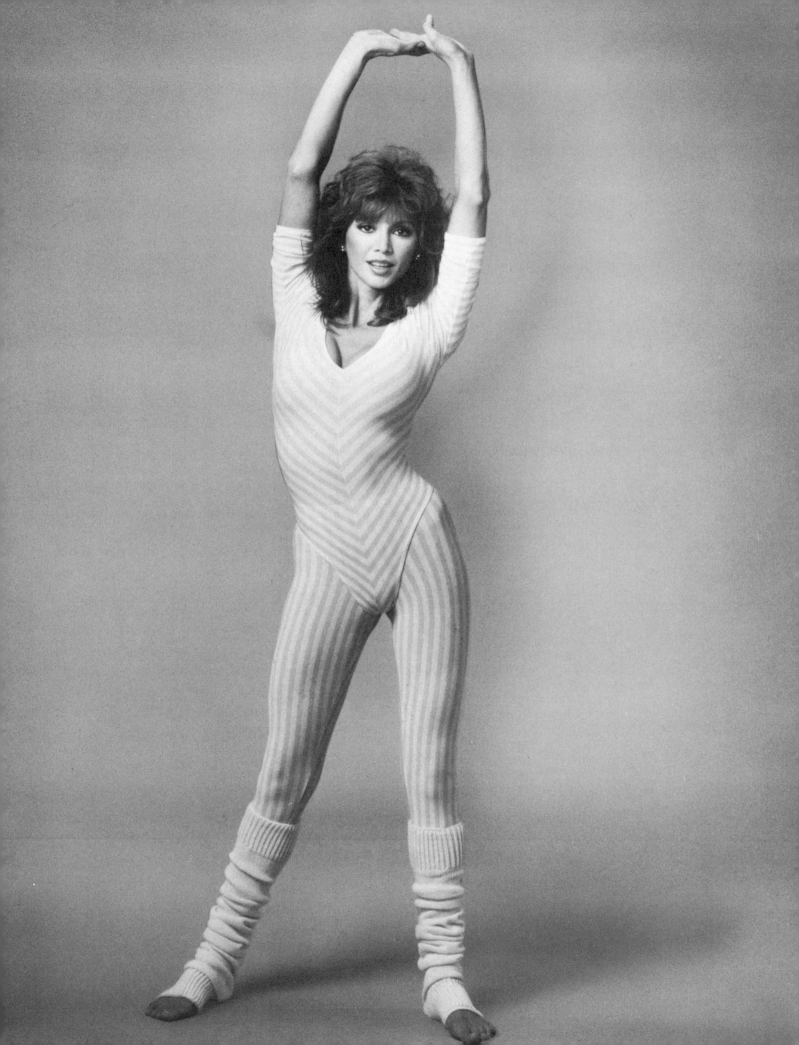

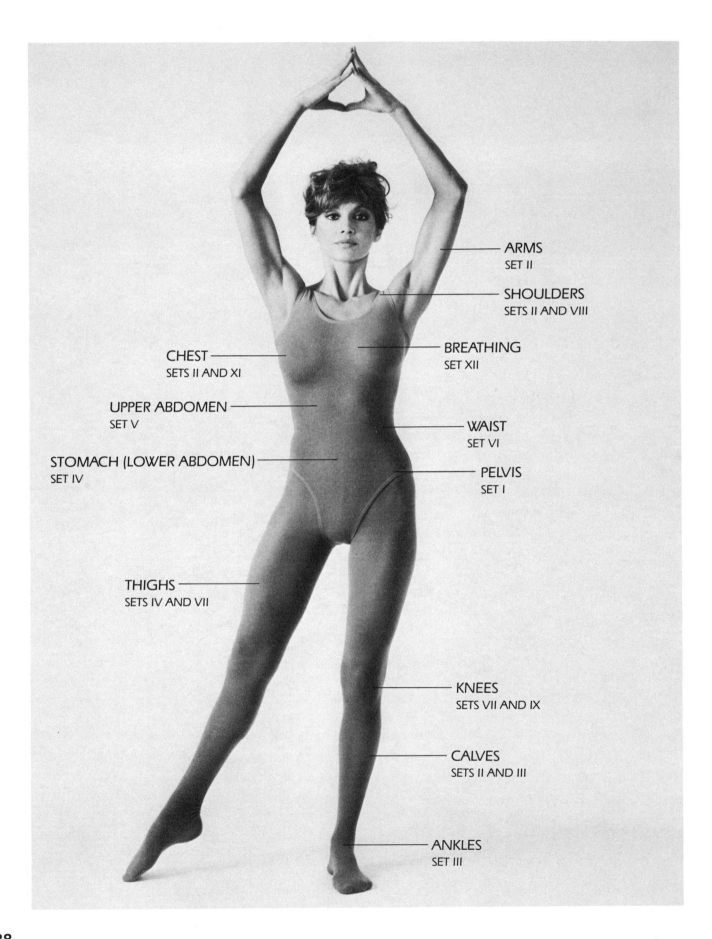

ARMS
SET II

SHOULDERS
SETS II AND VIII

BREATHING
SET XII

CHEST
SETS II AND XI

UPPER ABDOMEN
SET V

WAIST
SET VI

STOMACH (LOWER ABDOMEN)
SET IV

PELVIS
SET I

THIGHS
SETS IV AND VII

KNEES
SETS VII AND IX

CALVES
SETS II AND III

ANKLES
SET III

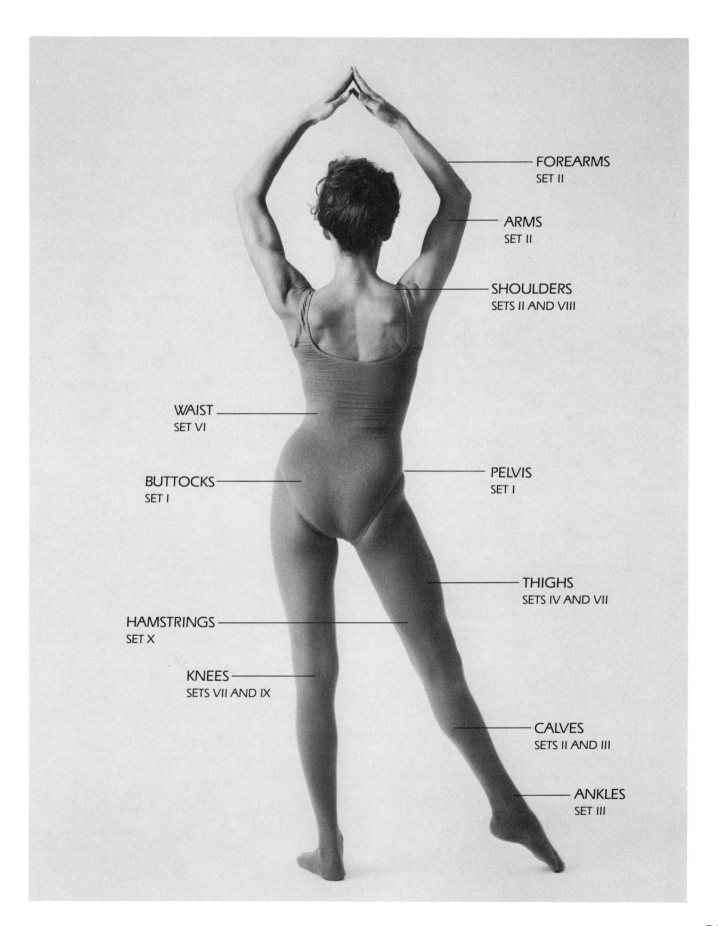

FOREARMS
SET II

ARMS
SET II

SHOULDERS
SETS II AND VIII

WAIST
SET VI

PELVIS
SET I

BUTTOCKS
SET I

THIGHS
SETS IV AND VII

HAMSTRINGS
SET X

KNEES
SETS VII AND IX

CALVES
SETS II AND III

ANKLES
SET III

in building up your arm muscles. Forget the exercise for the arm muscles and put together your own routine with the exercises for the buttocks, calves and thighs. List these exercises (leaving the optionals for when you are proficient at the regulars and/or have extra time to exercise), add up the time it takes to do each one (or each set), and you'll have the total concentrated time you'll need to exercise *(don't forget the warm-ups)*. Remember, you can add or subtract an exercise depending on its importance to you and the time it takes to do it (if you subtract one exercise, it could be the one you do in the car on the way to work or in the office later on in the day). The temptation is to try to do it all. Don't! My advice is to stick to the original time frame you decided on—you can always expand later. If you try to add more exercises immediately, chances are they will be too much for you and the whole program will suffer. The goal here is simplicity, because if the routine gets too complicated, you won't do it. And remember—when you finish your routine try to do a couple of stretches to cool down.

Once you learn how to do the exercises (and most are easy), the routine will become a part of your life. As you're driving to work, you'll do the exercises for the thighs. As you're sitting at the movies, you'll do the toe lifts for your calves. The beauty of my program is that you can be *so* flexible in both how much time you spend on each exercise, which ones you pick, and where you do them. No running to class, no doing exercises you don't need to do, no feeling guilty if you don't always have the time. It's convenient, easy, immediately effective—and a lot of fun.

Now, go to it!

THE BODY PRINCIPAL PROGRAM *

Set Number	Set Name	Number of Exercises	Time They Take	Where You Can Do Them
Set I	Warm-ups Buttocks & Pelvis	5 1	4 minutes ½ minute (or more; can repeat during the day)	On a firm bed; on a mat on the floor Standing (waiting in line anywhere); sitting in a chair (at the movies, in the car, at a beauty salon or at home waiting for hair to dry, talking on the telephone, taking a shower, vacuuming, etc.)
Set II	Arms, Forearms, Shoulders & Chest	2	1–2 minutes	At kitchen or bathroom counters; at a desk in the office
Set III	Calves & Ankles	3	2½ minutes	#1—On the stairs; #2—sitting in a chair (watching television, drying your hair, riding in a car)
Set IV	Stomach (lower Abdomen) & Thighs	2	1½ minutes	On a firm bed; on a mat on the floor
Set V	Upper Abdomen	1	¾ minute	On a mat on the floor
Set VI	Waist	2	1 minute	Standing at home or at the office with room to move
Set VII	Thighs	2	3½ minutes	On a mat on the floor
Set VIII	Shoulders	1	½ minute	Anywhere; perfect in the shower
Set IX	Knees	2	1 minute	Sitting in a chair; on a mat on the floor
Set X	Hamstrings	1	1 minute	On a mat on the floor or on the bed
Set XI	Chest & Breasts	1	¾ minute	At home or at the office
Set XII	Breathing	1	¾ minute	Anywhere, any time
	Warm-down (Warm-ups #2 & #3)	2	1½ minutes	Anywhere (in some privacy)

Total Time: Approximately 20 minutes

*This chart does not include the optional exercises; and all times are approximate. The Body Principal Program should be practiced daily, at one sitting or at various times throughout the day. If you want to put together your own program, see instructions in Chapter 2.

Warm-ups

You would think that everyone in the world knows you have to warm up before you exercise. But many people forget, or they figure they don't really need to. You should warm up each and every time you begin even the shortest of exercise routines. Even though it is almost impossible to hurt yourself with these resistive exercises, you may be uncomfortable and feel strained if you don't loosen up first. If you don't warm up you may do your exercises halfheartedly because your body is not flexible and your energy is low.

All exercise experts agree that it is essential to warm up before you attempt any exercise routine. According to Dr. Paul Ward, Director of Education, Research, and Development, Health and Tennis Corporation of America, warming up increases body and muscle temperatures (contraction and reflex times are improved with higher muscle temperatures), which increase energy production. In addition, warming up increases the blood and oxygen flow to the active muscles and also reduces stress on the heart and the likelihood of injury to soft tissue and muscles. So you can see how important it is to warm up (and warm down after finishing your exercise routine).

Once you do these simple warm-ups, you'll feel motivated—even eager—to begin your individualized exercise routine. You'll feel ready to exercise. Even if you get up one morning and realize that you won't have twenty minutes to do your exercises (you'll just have to do them at some other time in your day), it is still a good idea to take the three minutes to warm up so that your cardiovascular system is stimulated and you feel ready to take on the world. So, make it a rule: Do your warm-ups *before* you brush your teeth. It is a habit that is easy to develop.

Warming up is primarily stretching. When we stretch, one muscle is contracting and another is stretching. For example: While you are contracting your thigh muscles, the backs of your thighs (the hamstrings) are stretching. Thus, every time you do a stretch in your warm-ups, some muscles in your body are contracting, or tightening, and some are stretching, or extending. Keep in mind that during warm-ups you need only to concentrate on stretching your muscles, because they will contract naturally.

I start doing my warm-ups before I get out of bed. Doing a stretch (or any exercise, for that matter) on the bed (preferably one with a firm mattress) is a great way to avoid injuring yourself. That is because, when stretching on the floor, most of us will automatically arch our backs, which can result in a back injury.

WARM-UPS TIME: Approximately 4 minutes

NOTE: Don't check your watch every time you finish one of these steps. Do as much of a set as you think you need for approximately the stated time. After a few days, you'll automatically know when you have done enough and are ready to go on to the next step. Also remember: How much warming up you will need depends on what time of the day you are doing the warm-ups. In the morning, you may need more warming up than at lunchtime, when you have already spent half a day moving and stretching naturally.

WHERE: Do your warm-ups on your bed or on the mat on the floor of the bedroom, the office or wherever you are starting your routine. Remember: At home, try to do them without any clothes on except for the running exercise. (Here you will need a bra—or if you insist on not wearing one, hold up your breasts for support.) Obviously, at the office this may be difficult; so take off your shoes and, if possible, support hose or panty hose. If you can, turn on some music. I suggest you do these warm-ups in the order they are listed here. It has made sense for me, and I think it might work well for you. However, don't hesitate to change that order if it is more comfortable for you.

WARM-UP #1

After you wake up, take a few seconds to open your eyes, greet the day, smile if you feel like it, and get ready to start moving. Stretch your body as far as you can. Spread your legs, stretch your hands and arms back and up to the headboard of the bed, and stretch again. Reach as far as you can. Really feel your whole body move, slowly, almost like a cat. Stretch your fingers—agility in the fingers is very important. Feel the muscles in your shoulders and pelvis. Keep moving, slowly and easily. Stretch sensually, noting each movement of your muscles. Feel those muscles moving; feel the stretch down to your knees, your calves, your ankles, then your toes. Point your toes, curl them down, flex them up, and curl them again. Curl your fingers—now flex. Do your toes again. Curling your toes makes you use the muscles in your legs, thus resulting in noticeable definition of the fronts of the legs. Arch your body; arch it some more, moving leisurely, never jerking your body, just stretching every inch of it. When you think your body is all stretched out, stretch it one more time. Now you should feel your energy level rise.

This should take only 15 seconds.

Repetitions: 2

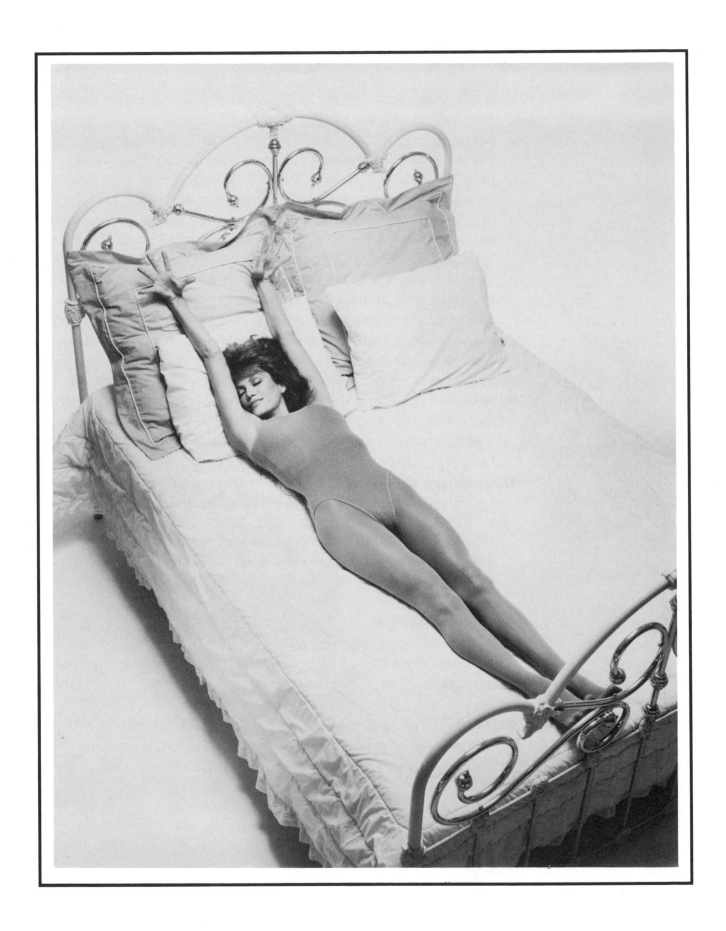

WARM-UP #2

1. Stand on the floor, feet flat (about 6 inches apart), heels on the floor, arms raised straight up.

2. Keep your knees bent (just a little) and try to touch the floor. I generally don't touch the floor my first few tries—so don't try to be a hero. Relax. Reach down; just hang over your body and wait. Hanging is great: When you hang, you don't arch your back, so the pressure on that area is released. You are stretching the muscles in your lower back, turning your pelvis and stretching your hamstrings. In fact, you are using a group of muscles you probably never even knew were there. Keep hanging, feel the muscles stretching in the back of your legs, through your thighs, in your buttocks, down your back, across your shoulders, to your fingertips. Keep hanging. (If you have a tendency toward back problems, try to keep your knees bent. Even those of us with so-called "lower-back problems" can warm up this way as long as the knees are bent). Do not tighten any muscles; just relax.

3. Now start exerting some force—reach toward the floor, then try to touch it. Push against the floor if possible until you feel your fingertips and hands beginning to support some of your weight. Stretch and hang—if you need to, keep your knees bent.

4. If you can, grasp your ankles and push your forehead toward your bent knees. The ultimate goal, once this becomes a daily habit, is to touch your forehead to your knees. When you can do this, you'll know you are truly stretched out—and you should congratulate yourself. If you can't touch your knees, don't get upset; that will be a goal to look forward to.

This should take 1 minute.

Roll up slowly to a count of 8 from the hanging position and get ready for the next warm-up.

NOTE: If you have a tendency toward a weak back, before coming back up from the hanging position, go down to a squat, put your hands on your knees and push against your knees to stand up.

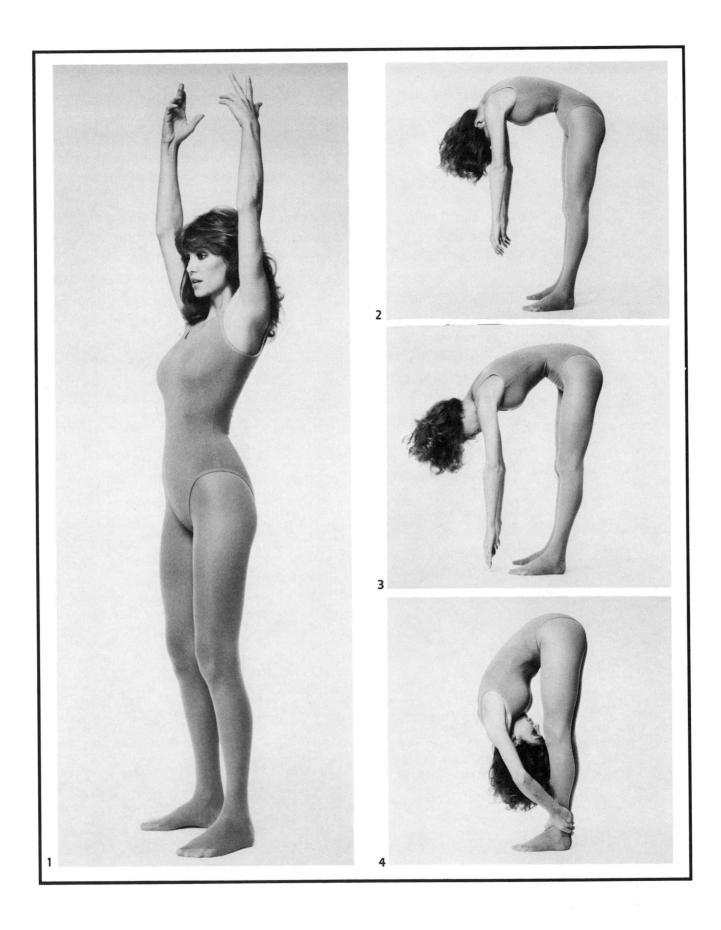

1

2

3

4

WARM-UP #3

Stand tall and loose with your feet a few inches apart, arms hanging straight down.

1. Roll your neck slowly to one side, trying to get your ear to touch your shoulder; then in one smooth movement roll toward the other side.
2. Come to center again and roll your neck forward and then up.

Do steps 1 and 2 four times consecutively. *Never* roll your head backward—that's tantamount to giving yourself a whiplash! There is no benefit to moving your head backward—and you really could hurt yourself. This exercise, done any time during the day, is also excellent for releasing tension and stress.

This should take 30 seconds.

Repetitions: 4

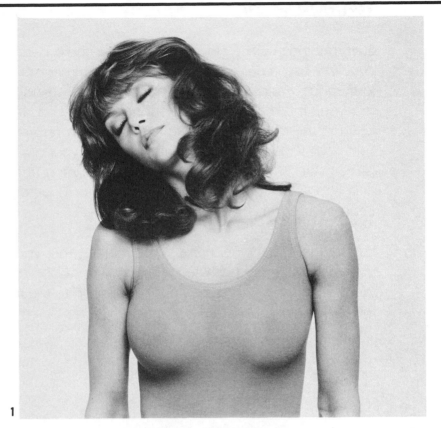

1

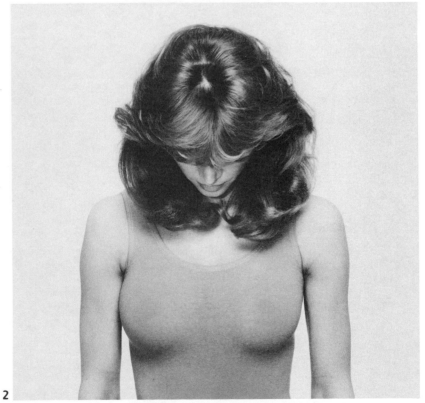

2

WARM-UP #4

Start running in place, slowly at first. This is the only deliberate cardiovascular exercise in our daily program (although many of the exercises exert just enough force to release enough energy to make your heart rate increase). It takes time to get your heart going, so start running slowly, keeping the momentum going (don't even stop to answer the phone). Your body temperature will also rise a bit, and your circulation will increase (speed up). When you feel your heart pounding (this usually happens after about 2 minutes), start slowing down for 15 seconds and then stop. Bend over to stretch your leg muscles.

Running in place should take you 2 minutes, but you can run longer if you wish. Now get ready to either move on to the next warm-up or, if you feel sufficiently stretched out, go right on to the first set of exercises in your chosen routine.

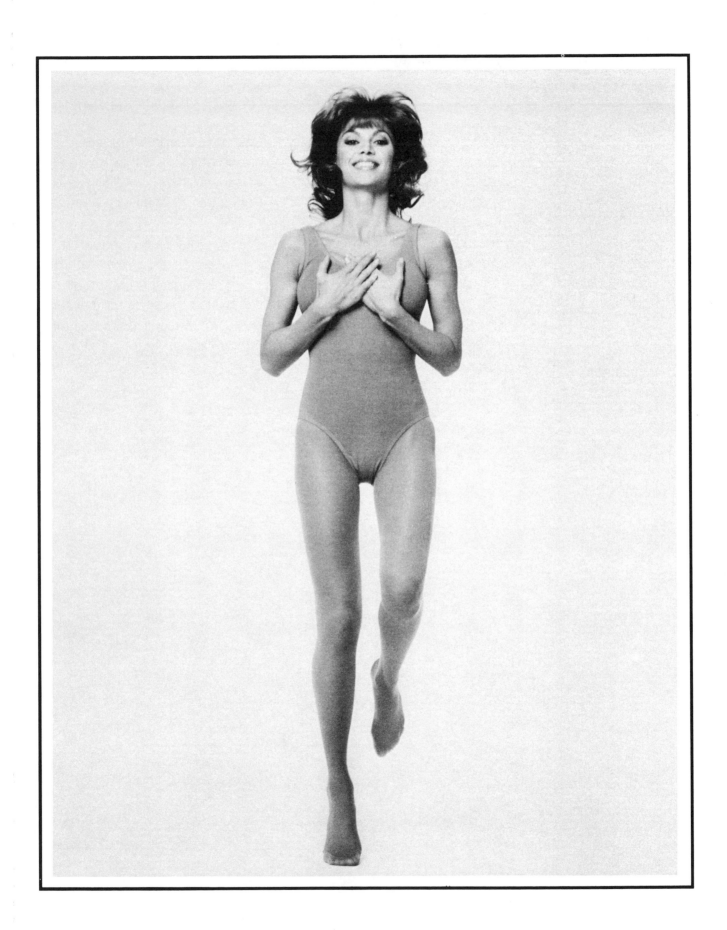

WARM-UP #5

1. Lie flat on your back on the floor (or on your mat), feet together, toes pointed.
2. Bring both knees up toward your chest. Hold for a moment. This movement alone—simple as it is—is one of the best things you can do for your back, because as soon as you bend your knees the pressure is off it. Do this movement once before and once after you do step 3.
3. Then straighten your legs flat on the floor, put your hands behind your head and pull your chin toward your chest very slowly (as long as you are comfortable); then back down, then up, then down again. Do this 8 times (what you are doing is lifting your head 8 times). Please remember you are not trying to give yourself a neck adjustment when you do this. Relax and stretch.

This should take no more than 30 seconds.

Repetitions: 8

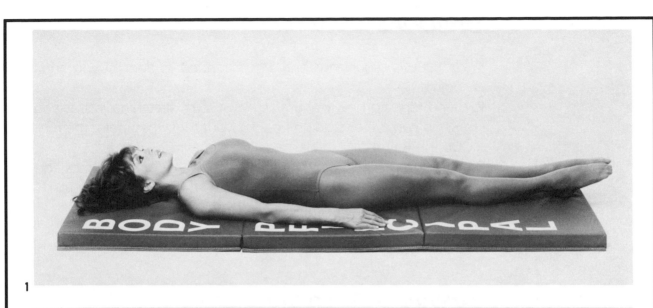

1

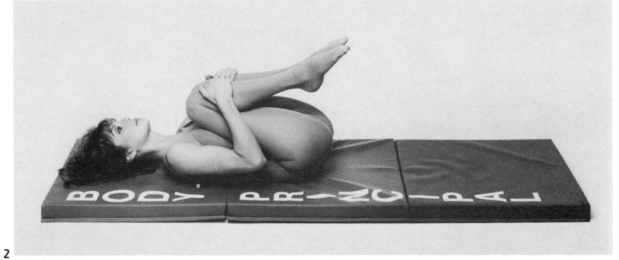

2

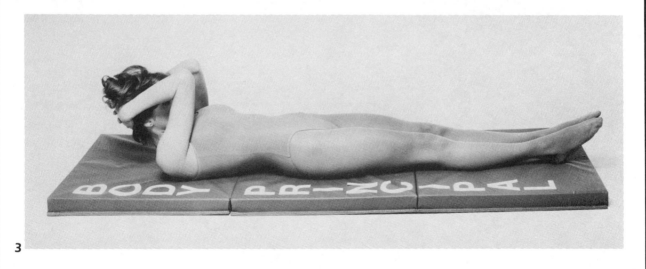

3

OPTIONAL WARM-UP

1. Sit up with your arms and legs extended in front of you and toes pointed.
2. Bend forward slowly and grasp your toes, stretching just as you did when you were standing up. Flex your toes, then point them again. Do this 8 times.
3. Then, if possible, point and flex your toes a few more times and see if you can get your forehead to touch your knees. Try it again. Now give up—and get up, and get ready to exercise.

This should take you 30 seconds.

Repetitions: 8 of step 2

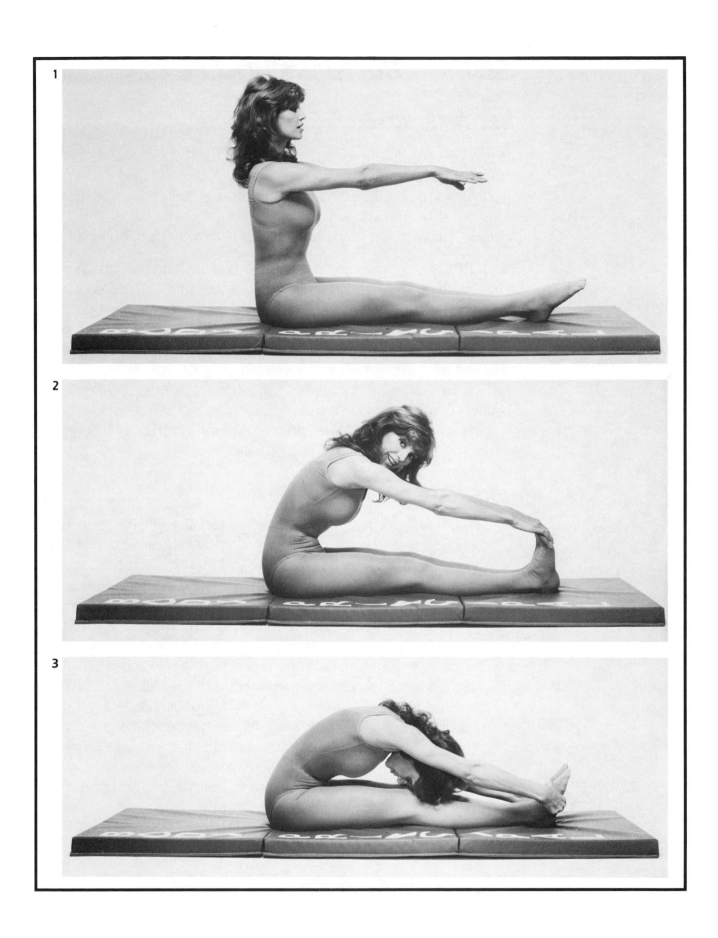

SET 1—Buttocks and Pelvis

SET TIME: 30 seconds to 1 minute

When you first do this exercise, you'll say, "Ooh, it's so simple!" You're right! But it is the perfect exercise. By tightening and releasing the buttocks (your bottom) and the pelvic muscles (you are contracting the stomach muscles also), you are toning your entire pelvic area and lifting your derrière. (You are also strengthening your back muscles considerably.)

WHERE: This exercise can be done standing or sitting in a straight, hard chair, pushing your back against the back of the seat. You can do it while waiting in line anywhere: at the movies or at the supermarket checkout counter. (However, watch your movements there: If others in line begin to move away from you, it may be a sign that you're moving too much.) You can do these while you are putting on your makeup, having your hair or nails done (do try to keep still while she is polishing), getting a suntan, vacuuming, taking a shower, driving a car or sitting on an airplane, reading, or talking on the telephone. You can do this set of exercises almost anywhere under any circumstances.

EXERCISE

1. Stand with your feet 12 inches apart, feet flat on the floor, knees slightly bent, (preferably in front of a mirror, at least at the beginning—this way you can watch every move you make).
2. Tighten the buttocks and the fronts and backs of the thighs, pull in your stomach, hold and release. Just let your hands drop at your sides comfortably. Learn to feel your muscles move. The rest of your body is relaxed; the only tightening that occurs is from your waist down. Try this to rhythmic music if you can; tighten again and release. Start out by doing 50 rapid movements. Yes, I did say 50. It is easier and takes less time than you may think, and you will notice a difference in your muscle tone in one week. As you get better at these, as they become somewhat automatic movements that you do everywhere you go, you will be able to do them more slowly. My rule is: A slow 50 equals a fast 100. Remember—this exercise can be done just as easily and effectively while you are sitting.

This takes 30 seconds if done quickly, 1 minute if slowly.

Repetitions: 50 to 100

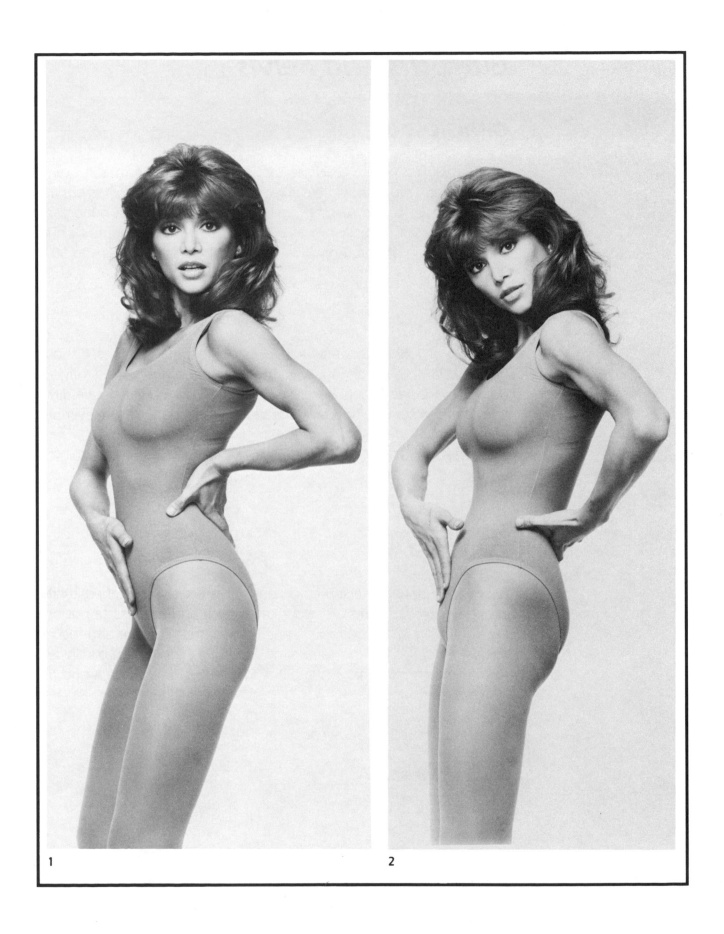

1 2

Buttocks and Pelvis

OPTIONAL #1

Another variation of this exercise is to tighten the same muscles while you are lying on the floor (preferably on a mat or a towel). In this position your contractions and stretches will tighten and tone your buttocks so that your bottom actually moves up higher to where it should be. This exercise should give you my ideal—"the bubble butt." Again do 50 to 100 movements as above.

This takes 30 seconds.

Take note of your bottom after a week of doing these exercises. It should be tighter and higher than it was. The more often and consistently you do these, the faster and better your results will be. Watch carefully—you'll be on your way to having the best "bubble butt" you've ever had.

Repetitions: 50 to 100

OPTIONAL #2

After you've done the first Buttocks and Pelvis exercise described, try this optional exercise. Stand with your knees bent and emphasize not only the tightening of the buttocks and the pelvic muscles, but also rocking the pelvis forward at the same time. You'll find you can naturally and without much effort move the pelvis forward. Back and forth—do this 50 times.

This should take 30 to 45 seconds.

Repetitions: 50

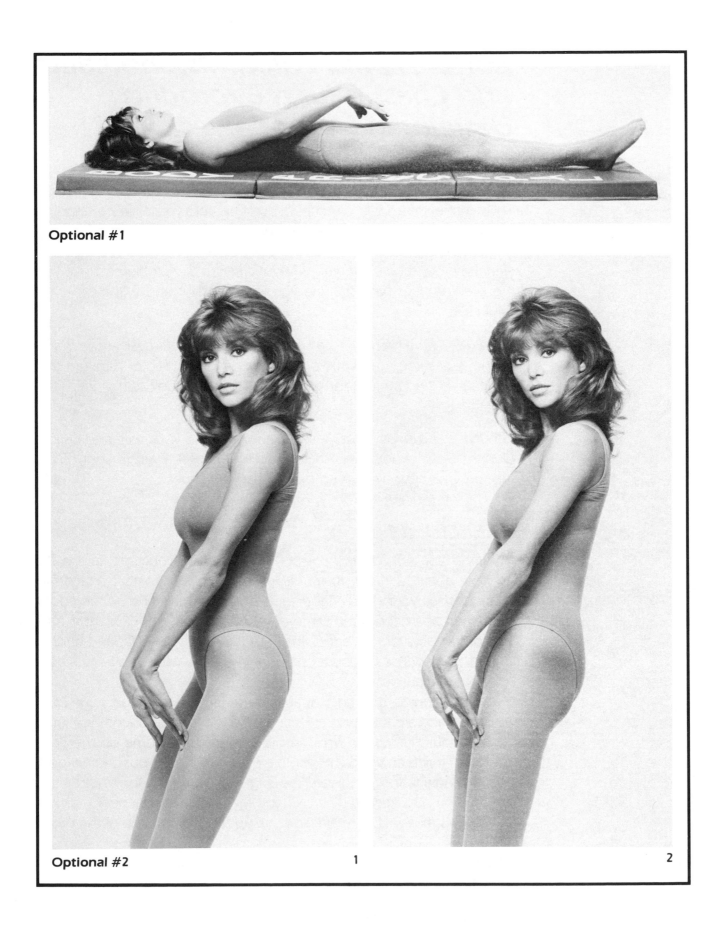

Optional #1

Optional #2

1

2

SET II—Arms, Forearms, Shoulders and Chest (Plus a Byproduct: Developing Your Calves)

SET TIME: 1 minute

This set of exercises is just like doing push-ups, but you do them standing up. They are much more effective than conventional push-ups. Doing these exercises standing builds up your pectoral and chest muscles and stretches your shoulder region without creating any problems. Since you are keeping your back straight, you won't arch it and will avoid back injuries.

WHERE: At the kitchen or bathroom counter, at your desk at the office, in the ladies' room at work, or at any stationary piece of furniture that appears to be about waist high (make sure it won't fold under your weight).

HINTS: Stand on a nonslippery surface so that your feet don't slide. Don't wear socks or hose—being barefoot is best. Even in your office, take off your hose or, if you can't, at least your shoes.

EXERCISE #1

1. Stand about 2 feet in front of a counter with your feet flat on the floor, about 12 inches apart. Without bending your knees, lean forward and place your hands flat on top of the counter (just at the edge), spread apart about the same distance as your feet. Hold your back completely straight; your stomach muscles must be tight and held in. Do not tighten the buttocks or any part of your body—just your stomach muscles.

2. Now, keeping that back straight and tummy in—drop your body slowly toward the counter until your chest almost touches it. Notice that your elbows are bent and your heels have come off the floor. Now straighten your arms completely, returning to your original position. Again—down toward the counter—and up. Don't hold either position, just keep moving smoothly. Make it a continuous down-and-up motion. Do 10 at first; work up to 25 by the end of the week.

Doing 10 should take 30 seconds. Doing 25 should take 1 minute, 15 seconds.

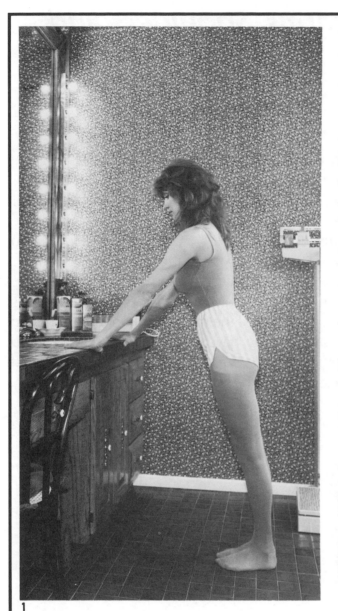

1

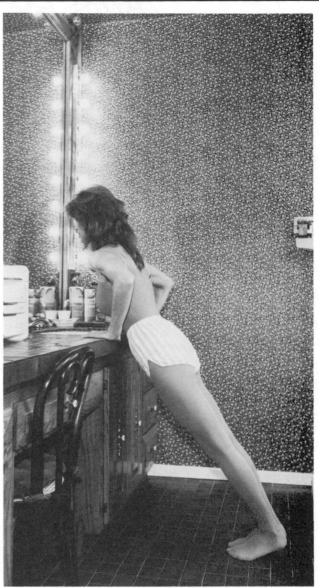

2

Repetitions: 10 to 25

Arms, Forearms, Shoulders and Chest

EXERCISE #2

1. Now try this exercise with your hands placed at the front of the counter, gripping the edge.
2. Drop toward the counter. Now return to your original position. This variation of the exercise is more stressful and makes use of still other muscles in your arms. Both Exercises #1 and #2 will develop your arm muscles and also stretch out your calves (that action happens when you are moving toward the counter and back). Please remember what I stressed in Chapter 2. This process of exercises uses resistance that will define and resculpt the muscles without making them bulge. Thus, whereas you may have never before thought about defining and strengthening your arm muscles, now you can do both without risk of developing bulging arms. Do 10 of these.

This should take 30 seconds.

Repetitions: 10

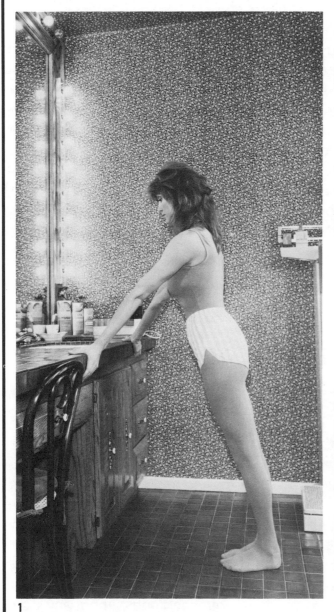

1

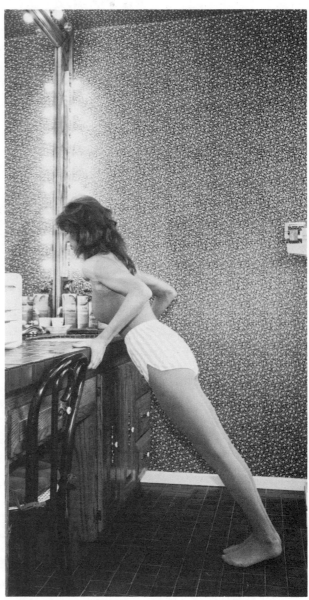

2

Arms, Forearms, Shoulders and Chest

OPTIONAL #1

Do this with your hands either on the top of the counter or at the front edge, but keep your *heels on the floor.* This is a terrific exercise because while you are toning the upper muscles and stomach, you are also stretching your calf muscles and the muscles that form your Achilles' tendon. (As a matter of fact, if you are interested in sculpting your calves more, you can go directly from this exercise to the one for the calves because your calf muscles will already be stretched out.) Do 10 at first, working up to 25 by the end of the first week. Stay at 25—you don't need to increase the number of times you do this exercise.

This takes 30 seconds.

Repetitions: 10 to 25

OPTIONAL #2

1. Stand sideways to the counter, placing one hand on top of it at the edge.
2. Keep your body straight and start moving toward the counter; return slowly, pushing your weight with your arm. Here you'll be using more chest muscles and developing your flank (the middle portion of the body). This exercise will also thin out your waist. It is a difficult movement because all your body weight is on one arm at a time. Do it slowly, 5 the first week, 10 the second, working up to 25 a day when you feel you can do them comfortably and without any strain. Repeat the exercise with the opposite arm.

Doing 5 should take 15 seconds. Doing 10 should take 30 seconds. Doing 25 will take at least 1 minute.

Repetitions: 5 to 25 each side

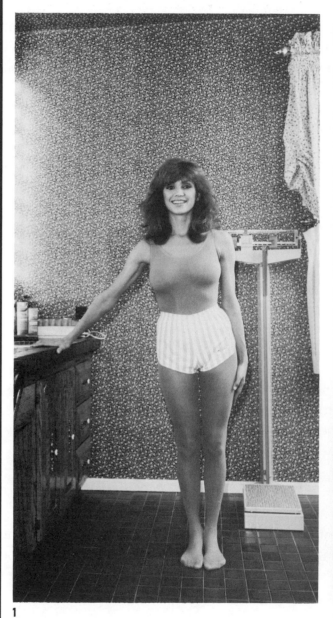

1

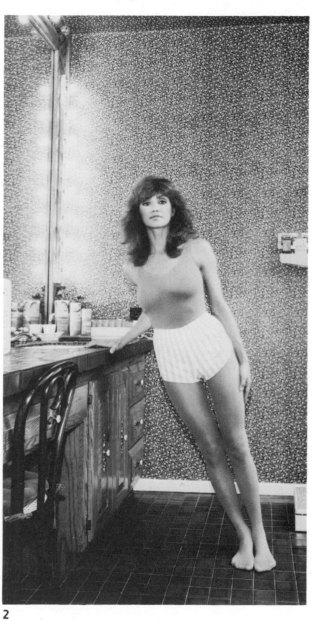

2

Optional #2

65

SET III—Calves and Ankles

SET TIME: 2 minutes, 30 seconds

Calves are my weakness. My calves, you should know, are a legend on the set of "Dallas." For years Patrick Duffy would greet me with, "Hey, Victoria, find your calves yet?" As a matter of fact, I've been late to work looking for my calves. But no more. I've been doing these exercises for three years and have developed (and kept) defined, noticeable and, to me, beautiful calves. Gone are the straight skinny legs. Hello shapes! And I noticed a difference after two weeks, which was a strong motivating factor in my zeal to find resistive exercises that have anything to do with calves. This set of exercises is so easy and so startlingly and obviously effective it will knock your socks off. I have since learned that most people have a difficult time developing the calves they want. Runners try, but what they get is tremendous strength and bigger muscles. That's not what I wanted—I wanted distinct, shapely calves. This exercise pinpoints the calf muscles and works on those that will resculpt the calf without creating larger, bulging muscles.

WHERE: Standing on the stairs (Exercise #1); sitting in a chair with a straight back or sitting on the stairs (Exercises #2 and #3). On the stairs be sure to sit up straight with your feet two steps below you so your thighs are parallel to the floor. If you can, watch the news or listen to music while you do them.

EXERCISE #1

1. Stand on a step (not the first one) on the balls of your feet, facing as if to go up the stairs. Make sure there is a banister or wall next to you for balance, not for support. Your heels are off the step, so your arches are *not* supported by anything except the balls of your feet.

(continued)

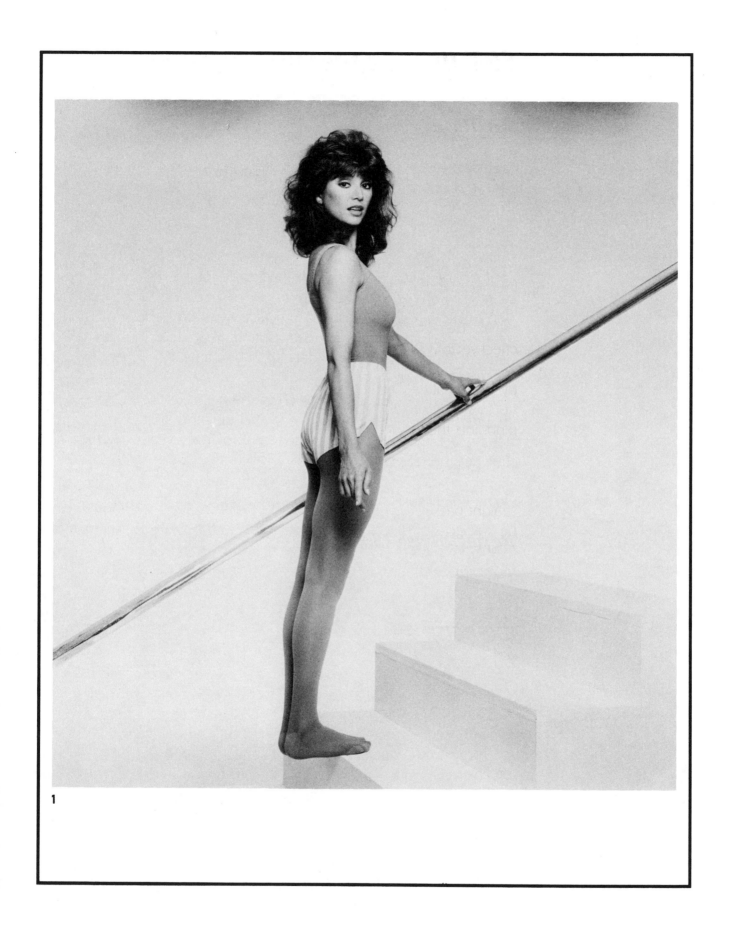

1

2. Raise yourself up on the balls of your feet.
3. Then drop your heels as far as you can below the step; now up again above the step and then to where you were before. Don't forget to breathe. Start by doing 25 and work up to doing 50. Keep going up and down—slowly. No jerking, just a smooth raising and lowering of the body, using only your feet, moving with great control.

Be sure your body is relaxed while you are doing this exercise. Don't tighten any muscles. Concentrate only on the smooth up-and-down movement. Don't push too hard. Calf muscles tend to get sore if you strain them. After a day or so, the soreness should go away, but you may confuse the pain with newly defined calf muscles. Forget it! Even my exercises won't give you new legs in one easy session! So work slowly— don't overdo, especially during the first week, as your entire body is getting used to its new exercise routine. Your new muscles will be perfectly (but not too largely) defined in due time. If you get tired, stop and flex your feet.

When you are done, go right on to the next exercise in this set. It is important to do the calf exercises one after the other; that's why I suggest starting the set for calves after the one for the forearms (which also stretches the calves).

Doing 25 will take about 1 minute.

Repetitions: 25 to 50

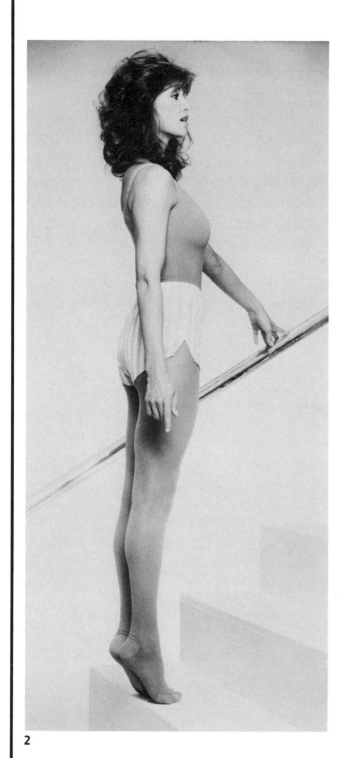

2

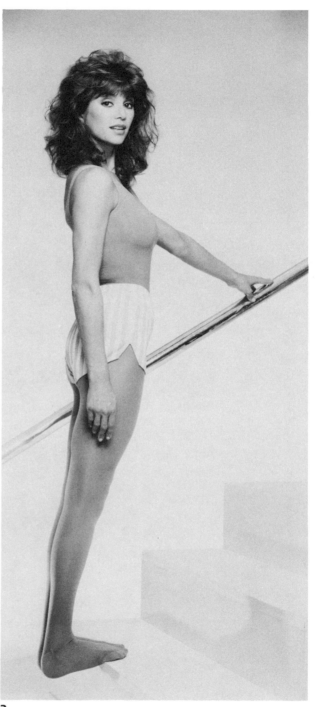

3

Calves and Ankles

EXERCISE #2

1. Sit on a chair with a firm back, feet flat on the floor.
2. Then do 50 toe lifts. Simple! Keep your heels on the floor for 25, (this should take about 30 seconds).
3. Next keep both the heels and the balls of your feet on the floor for another 25 (another 30 seconds). These lifts (they are also called "flexes" by some) will stretch out the calves and further redefine (or resculpt) them. This exercise will ensure that, if you have calves that fall toward the ankles, they will now stay where they belong. It will also strengthen your ankles. Keep relaxed in the chair; don't clench your neck or your shoulders. Keep lifting those toes. When you are done, stretch your legs out by walking around the room a couple of times, pointing your toes every now and then.

This takes 1 minute.

Repetitions: 25 each

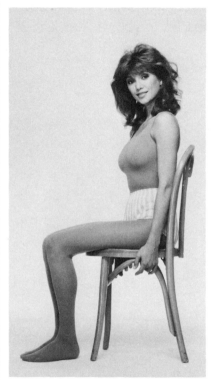
1

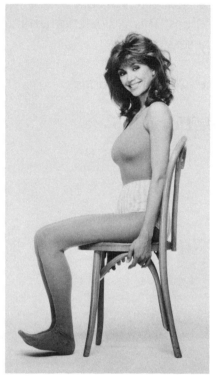
2

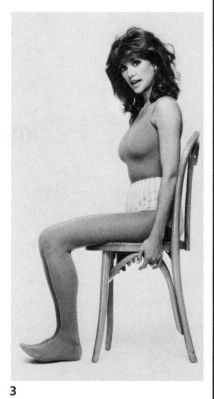
3

Calves and Ankles

EXERCISE #3

1. Stay seated in your chair. Place your feet flat on the floor, keeping your knees straight.
2. Then turn your feet out from the ankle, then back in. In and out, just like a duck. Keep in control—only the feet are moving in and out, not the knees. This will strengthen the muscles in your ankles. Do 25 at every session.

This takes 20 to 30 seconds.

Repetitions: 25

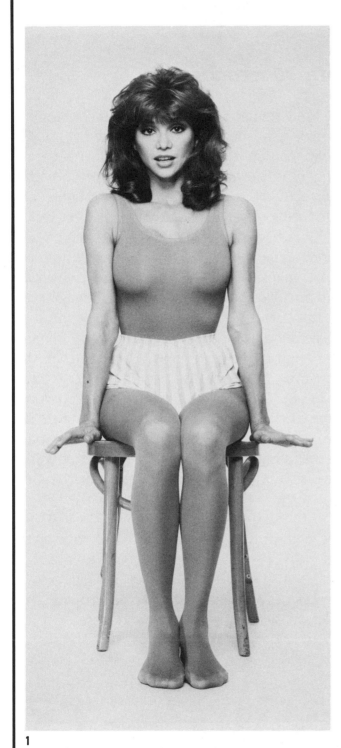

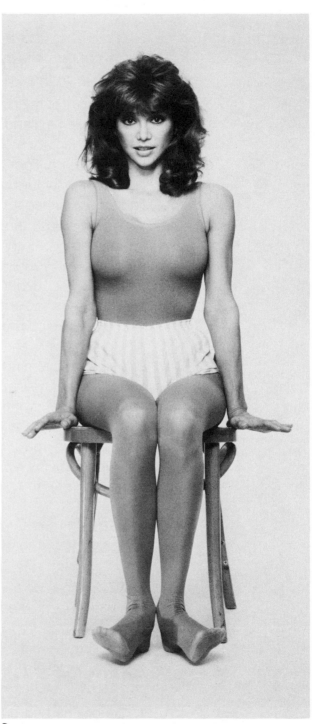

1

2

73

SET IV—Stomach (Lower Abdomen) and Thighs

SET TIME: 1 minute, 30 seconds

The nucleus of my figure is my stomach—I have a flat and tight tummy. (I once asked a friend of mine to hit me in the stomach with her fist. First she blanched; then she warmed up to the challenge and smacked me in the stomach. Poor thing—she really hurt her hand.) If your stomach is flat and tight, your bottom is usually going to be higher and tighter and your thighs firmer—not to mention that your lower back muscles will be stronger because those stomach muscles will take the pressure off your back. Imagine, all this from tightening your stomach! Your posture will be better, and your internal organs will fit better in your body, which will make you feel better. It's a terrific chain reaction. Follow the exercises and you'll see some results—fast.

In these exercises you are using all the muscles that hook on from the hip to the thigh and the thigh to the knee, plus again stretching the calves. Let me remind you: Every muscle that you contract on one side is stretching on the opposite side. Thus, as you are tightening your lower abdomen (the front), the backs of your legs are getting stretched. Contracting is the active, stretching is the passive movement. In other words, when you are consciously contracting (working) the abdomen and upper thighs, you are also, without deliberate effort, stretching the backs of the legs.

WHERE: These exercises for the lower abdomen should be done on the bed.

HINT: You can do these exercises after you do your first warm-ups when you wake up, provided you really feel stretched out and loose.

EXERCISE # 1

1. Lie on the bed on your back, your knees hooked over the side and your feet hanging down. Keep your hands at your sides.

(continued)

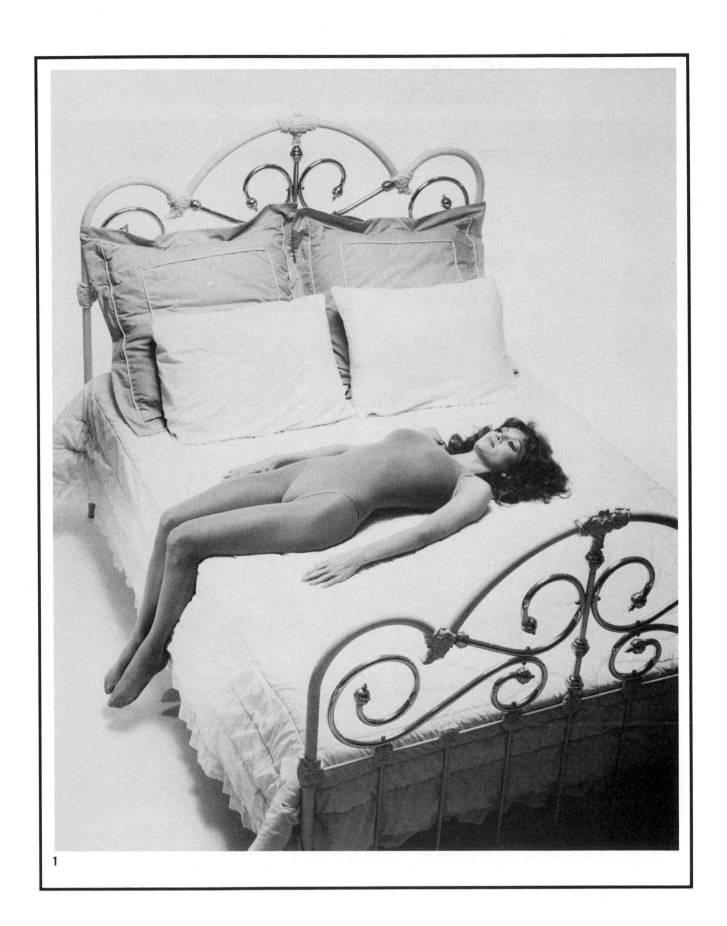

1

2. Slowly raise your legs from the floor until your knees are straight and your legs are parallel to the floor; then slowly bring them down again. What is happening here is you are toning the muscles in the front of your thighs and at the same time stretching your calves. Do 10 of these.

3. Next bring both knees to your chest to rest (similar to a hug). Now you are warmed up for Exercise #2 of this set.

This takes 20 to 30 seconds.

Repetitions: 10 of step 2

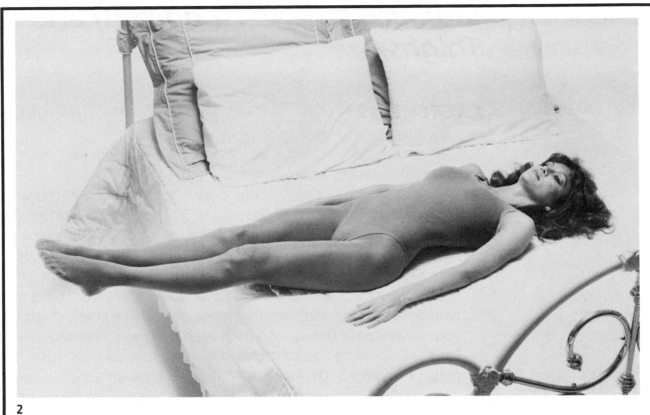

2

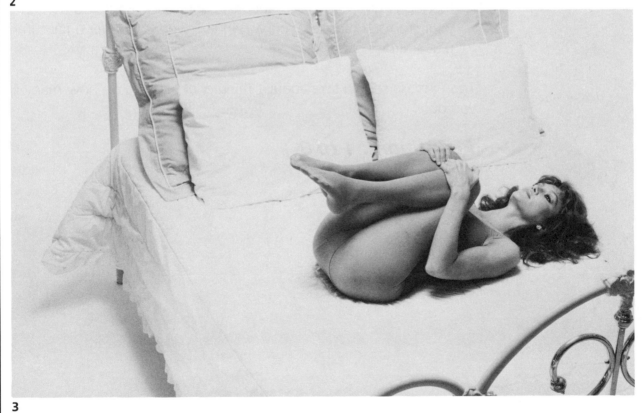

3

Stomach (Lower Abdomen) and Thighs

EXERCISE #2

1. Stay on the bed. Place your legs straight out in front of you, parallel to the floor—knees locked—and count to 4.
2. Then raise your legs slowly, keeping your knees straight, all the way up as high as you can while counting to 4 as you go. Keep breathing and lower your legs, still straight, to the count of yet another 4. (I never said this would be as easy as the other, did I?) Relax. . . . You only have to do this once the first morning (20 seconds), twice the next (30 seconds), and so on. But never do more than 8. This is the perfect exercise to tighten the thighs and at the same time strengthen your lower stomach muscles, which are the key to lower-back problems (plus—doing this on the bed ensures that you will have no pressure on your back). In reality, you should know that there is really no such thing as a weak back muscle—only weak stomach muscles that don't give adequate support to your back. So if you tighten up your stomach muscles, you win in every way; you get a flat tummy plus a strong back.

This exercise should take about 1 minute, depending on how many lifts you do.

Repetitions: 1 to 8

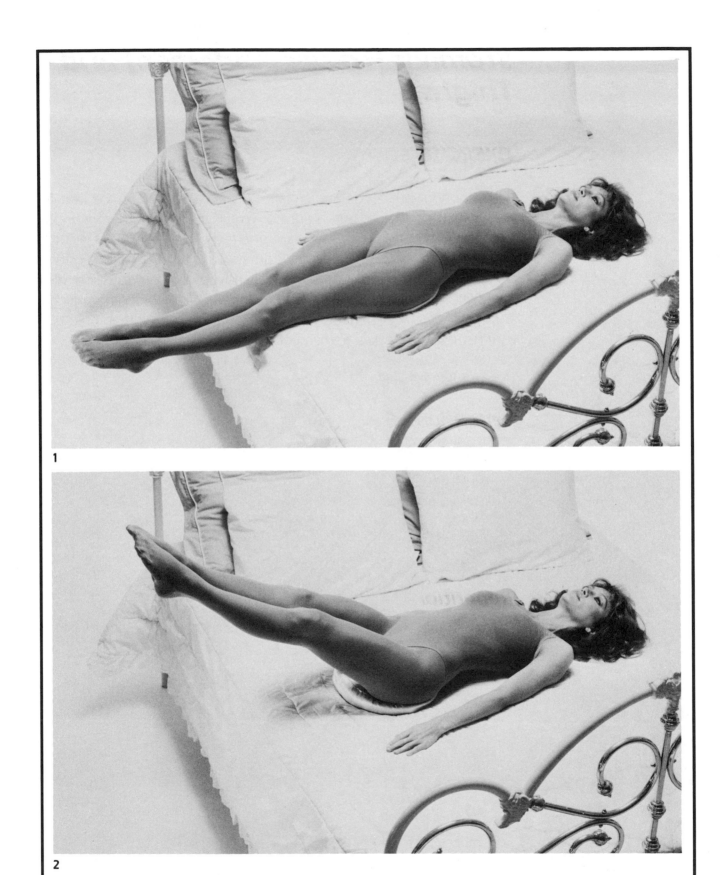

1

2

79

Stomach (Lower Abdomen) and Thighs

OPTIONAL

Do this when you can do the leg lifts 4 times easily. Stay on the bed on your back, legs straight out in front of you. Now, making a continuous scissors motion with both legs, raise them up to the count of 4, then down to the count of 4. Do this 8 times. It is hard but well worth it, because it again tones the abdominal muscles while tightening your thighs (exterior and interior), hip joints, the backs of your thighs (hamstrings) and your calves. It even helps your heart, because you work so hard that your heart rate increases. Remember to keep breathing normally.

This should take at least 1 minute.

Repetitions: 8

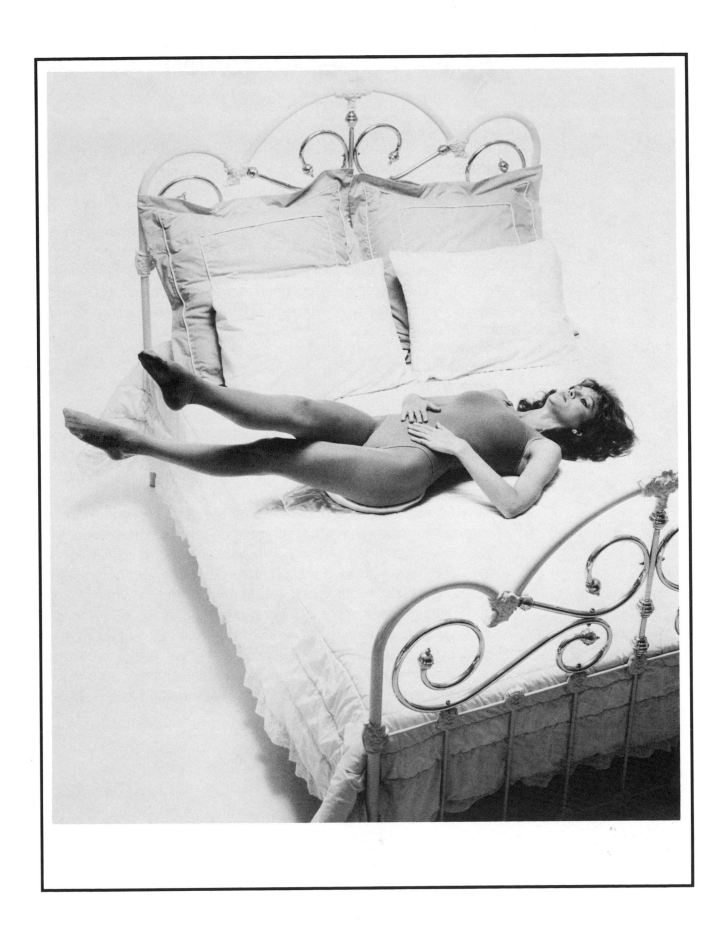

SET V—Upper Abdomen

SET TIME: 45 seconds

WHERE: On the floor at home or at the office—preferably on a clean surface. (Get a mat; you'll be able to use it for many exercises.)

HINT: When you are doing a sit-up and you raise yourself beyond the first 10 inches, those extra inches off the ground are only a waste of energy; they will not help your abdominal muscles. Most people yank as hard as they can on the neck and get minimal stomach activity. The only thing you should feel are your stomach muscles contracting, thereby lifting you up. That's all!

EXERCISE

1. Lie down on the floor, knees bent, feet flat on the floor. Place your fingertips on the tops of your shoulders, elbows pointed straight up (if you grasp your shoulders, you will jerk yourself up, and that's wrong).
2. Now lift your head and upper torso off the floor. Feel your stomach getting tight. Make sure you are coming up from the shoulders only— your lower abdomen is doing nothing. Keep your back flat against the floor. Now hold for a second, then down, up and down again. Be sure to breathe out when you come up and in when you go down (and remember my lecture on breathing; make loud noises to show yourself you are really working). Start with 20 repetitions, then work up to 50. Once you have reached 50 (it will take a week or so to be able to do that many and feel comfortable), there is no reason to do any more. Your upper abdomen will be getting all the tightening action it needs.

If you do twenty, it should take 45 seconds.

Repetitions: 20 to 50

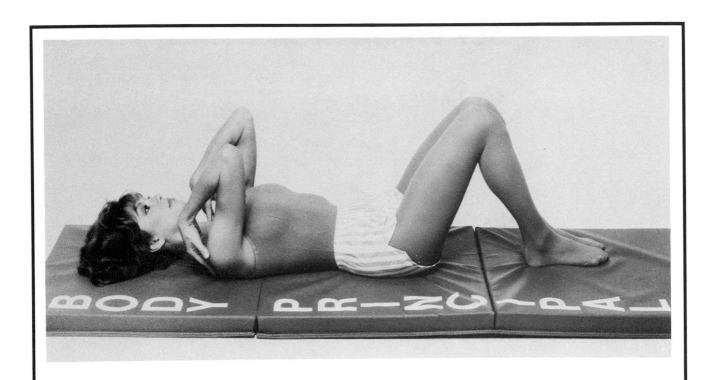

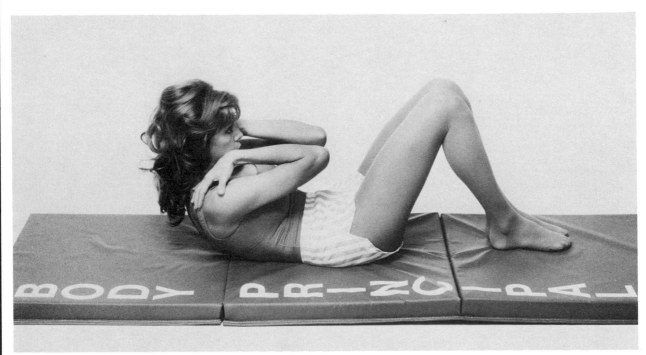

2

SET VI—Waist

SET TIME: 1 minute

WHERE: Wherever you have room to swing your arms and move comfortably without hitting anything.

EXERCISE #1

1. Stand straight, feet flat on the floor about 8 inches apart. Hold your arms straight out in front of you with hands clasped.
2. Bend forward from the waist and hang over.

(continued)

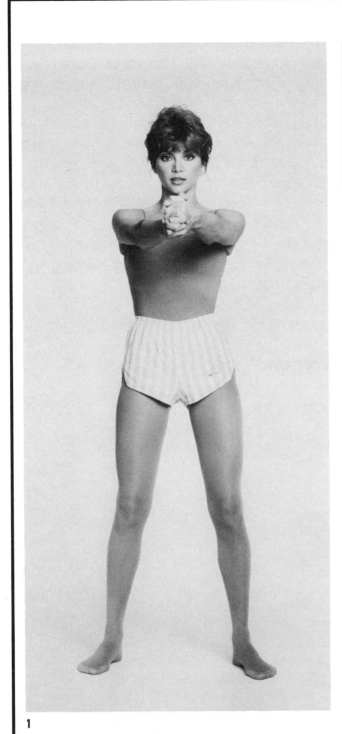

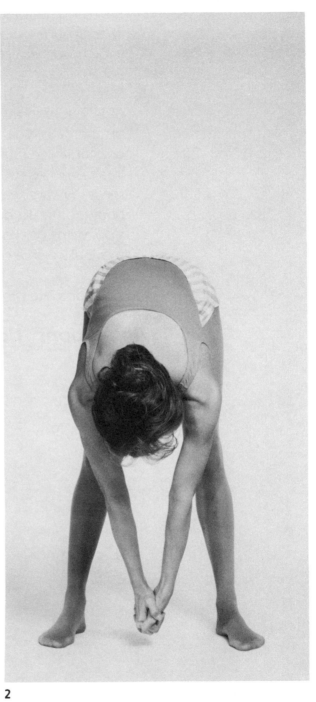

1

2

3. Then turn your body toward your left foot.
4. In a continuing motion, start moving up to a count of 8, holding your hands out in front of you, finishing with your hands on top of your head (you resemble the movements of the hands of a clock, with your head between your arms). Keep your buttocks and stomach tightened.
5. Stop when your hands are on top of your head and hold to a count of 8. Return to the first position. Now do the same exercise starting on the other side. Do not use force or momentum. The secret is to use controlled muscles. *Never* swing your arms or your body—move in a deliberate controlled action. (Even the stop is a controlled movement.) Always keep your head moving in the same direction as your body. You really do look like a clock; each movement is a start and stop, with your body moving smoothly. Don't tighten anything—just move along in a controlled motion.

Do one complete circuit to each side. This should take 30 seconds.

Repetitions: 1 circuit each side

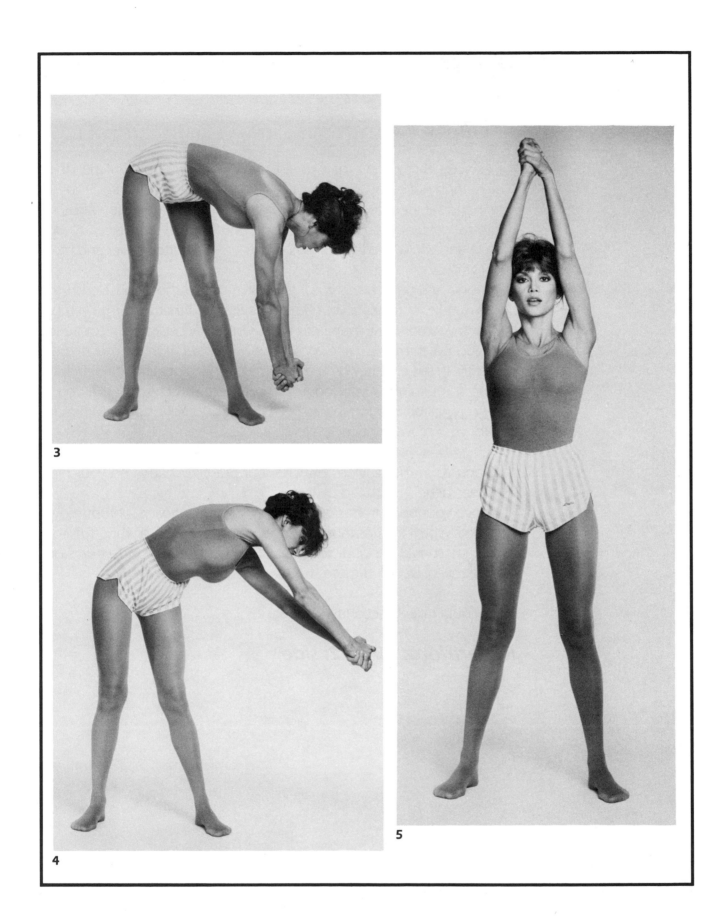

3

4

5

Waist

EXERCISE #2

An exercise that people have been doing for years to slim the waist which I find not particularly beneficial is to swing the body from side to side, hands at the waist. (Besides, you'd have to jerk from side to side for hours to get any results, and by then **you**'d have probably pulled a muscle and you'd surely be exhausted.) There is a better, easier and more effective way.

To tone and tighten the waist you have to use those muscles in the upper middle, or flank, of your body. I have found that with my method, in which you don't use momentum to twist or jerk but rather a controlled stop-and-go turn from side to side, the muscles tighten much more efficiently. In this exercise you use your upper and lower abdomen muscles to stop the turning of your body, for it is these muscles that put you in motion and stop you when you get to each side. Your stomach muscles control your movement completely.

1. Stand as in the previous exercise, but put your hands on your hips, knees bent.
2. Move your body from side to side in short, controlled, abrupt movements (you'll look as though you're doing a version of kung fu). Your breath should be audible, your movements short and your stops controlled. Do 20 of these (10 on each side).

This should take 30 seconds.

Repetitions: 10 each side

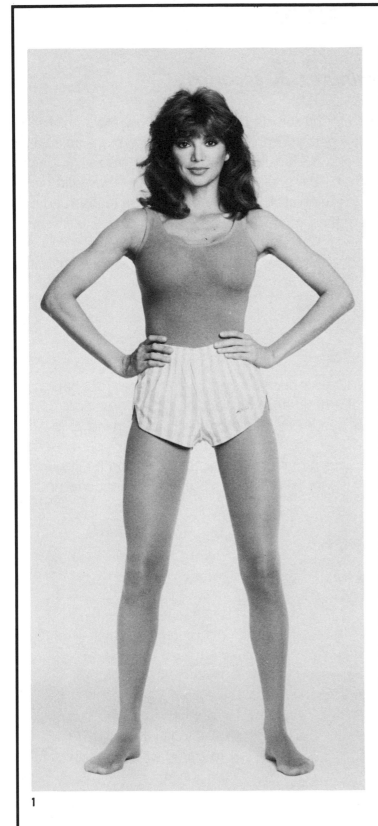

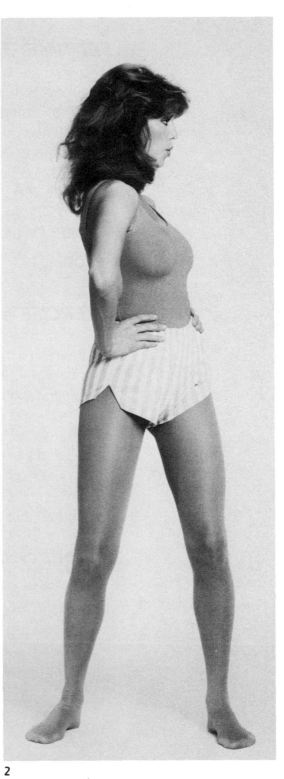

1

2

89

SET VII—Thighs

SET TIME: 3 minutes, 30 seconds

I was ecstatic when I found this simple exercise for my problem area—thighs. This is where I get a build up of fatty cells (some people call it cellulite). I can still feel some small fat deposits rolling around. Rub your hands up and down the backs of your thighs and feel those little rolls. Not much fun? Well, take heart. Those fatty cells will be reabsorbed into your body after you tighten and tone your thighs with these exercises.

WHERE: On the floor or a mat, at home or at the office. You can watch television as you do these exercises.

EXERCISE #1

Lie down on a mat with your heels pressed against a wall (or a stationary object like the side of a desk) and your legs at a 45-degree angle. Press against the wall with your heels as though you are trying to push it away from you (you'll see the muscle on the insides of your kneecaps coming toward you, which makes this exercise also good for tightening the knee). Hold for a count of 10. Do this 5 times, remembering not to hold your breath.

This should take 30 seconds.

Repetitions: 5

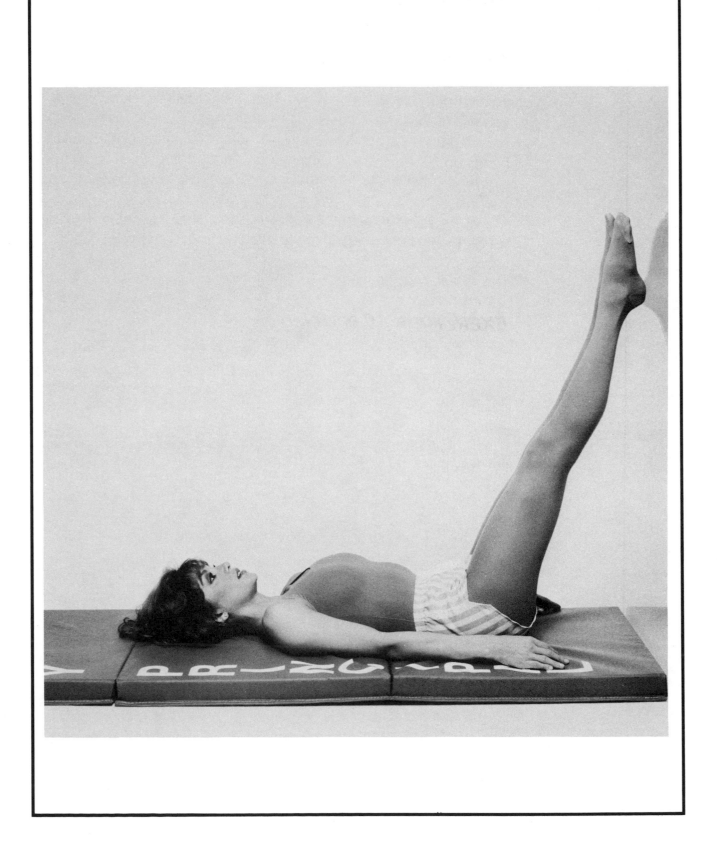

Thighs

EXERCISE #2

1. Stand in front of a mirror with both feet together. You will need to balance yourself—your fingertips on a chair or a desk will be fine. Lift one leg slowly to the side until it is horizontal (in the beginning, lift it up only as high as you can—it took me a while before I could make that horizontal lift). Now hold for a count of 10, lower slowly. Do 5 of these lifts.
2. Do the same thing to the front—lift, hold, then lower 5 times. Then repeat the exercise again to the side and front with the other leg.

This should take 3 minutes.

Repetitions: 10 each leg

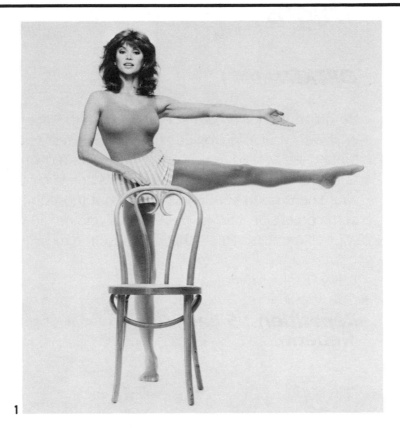

1

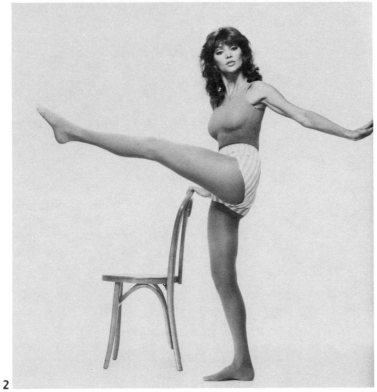

2

Thighs

OPTIONAL #1

Lie on your back on the floor or on a mat. Place your feet against the wall with your legs crossed at the ankles. Press your top leg against the bottom leg as hard as you can and hold for a count of 10. Do 5 times to start. This will take about 30 seconds. When you complete one side, pull your knees up to your chest, stretch out those thigh muscles, and then to the other side 5 times. This will take another 30 seconds. You may feel yourself tremble a little—that's because the muscles are contracting.

This will take 1 minute.

Repetitions: 5 each side

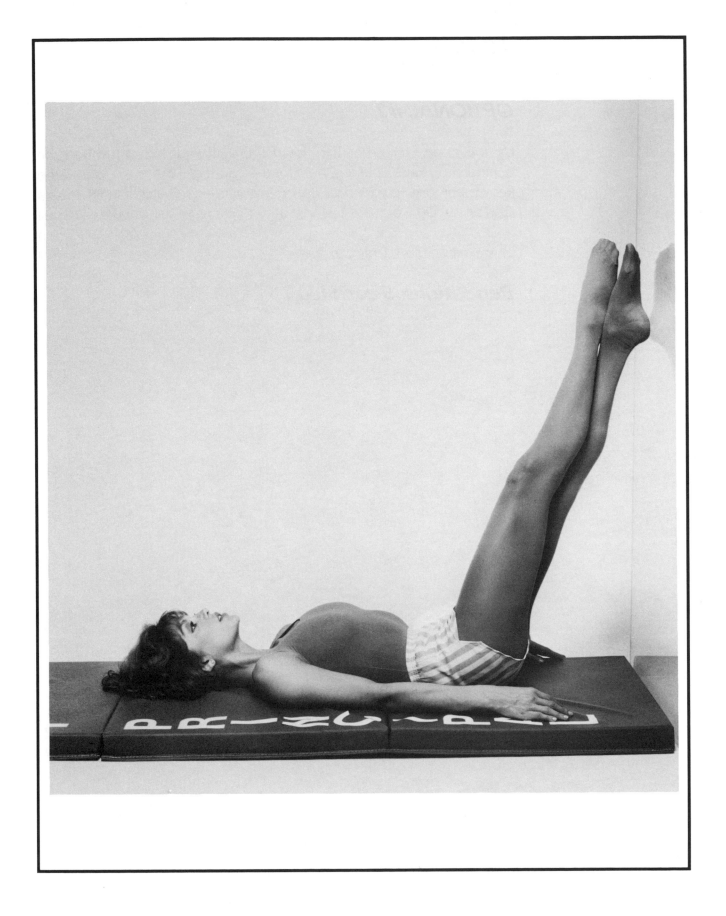

Thighs

OPTIONAL #2

Do the same exercise as Exercise #2, but lift your leg to the back (or behind you). Raise your leg, hold for the count of 10, then lower slowly. Remember to keep your back flat on this one—don't arch it or let it bow. Don't rush. Do 5 of these lifts and then repeat with the opposite leg.

This exercise takes 1 minute.

Repetitions: 5 each leg

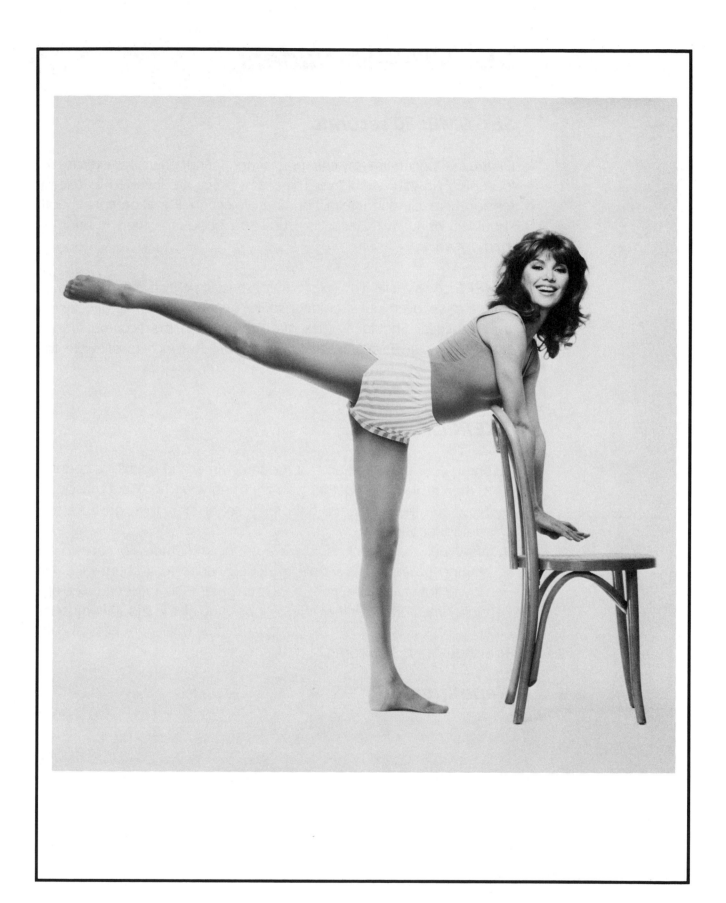

SET VIII—Shoulders

SET TIME: 30 seconds

Dr. Bruce Oppenheim (my chiropractor and friend) offers this exercise for loosening up your shoulders. Three easy steps are involved to release tension here: elevation, retraction and projection. Elevation entails both shoulders rising; with retraction, both go back. Projection is bringing them forward.

WHERE: Anywhere. This exercise is especially effective in the shower with a towel over your shoulders, so the heat can penetrate directly into the shoulders. Shoulder aches often result from the accumulation of tension in your daily life. This exercise will do much to alleviate that tension.

EXERCISE

1. Shrug your shoulders, both at the same time, and hold for a count of 1, then relax them together (you are using your rhomboid muscles).
2. Now curl them forward, hold for a count of 1, then go back to a straight position.
3. Now pull them back, hold for a count of 1, then go back to the starting position. The whole exercise is done to a count of 6. Up, down, forward, straighten, back, straighten. Do the entire set of 6 eight times, one after the other to loosen up all the shoulder muscles.

This should take 30 seconds.

Repetitions: 8

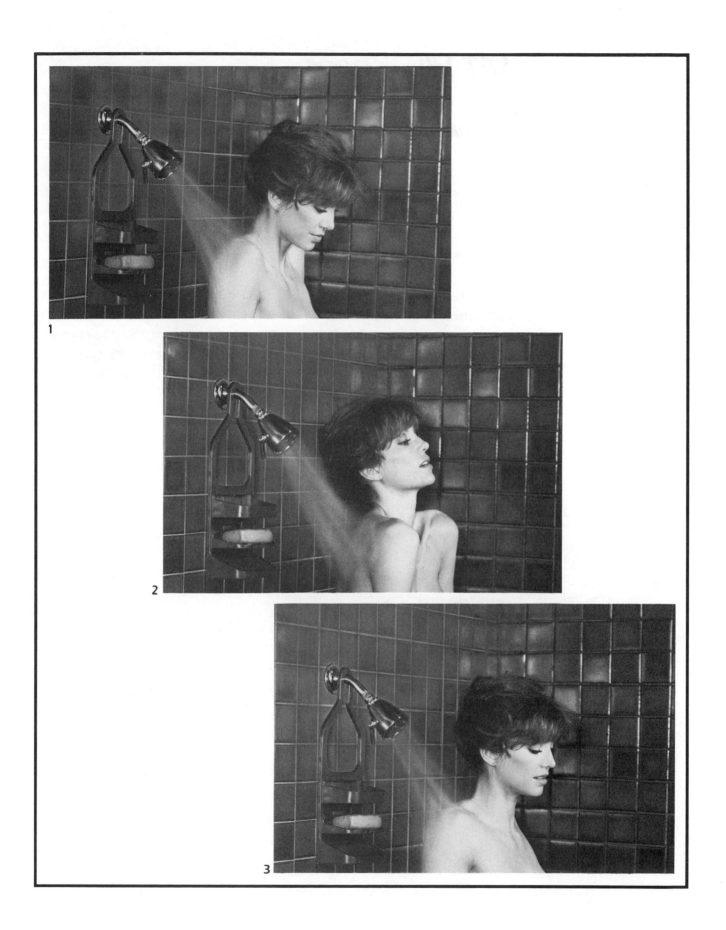

1

2

3

SET IX—Knees

SET TIME: 1 minute

WHERE: On a firm chair anywhere—try it at the movies. The second exercise is done on a mat on the floor.

EXERCISE #1

Sit up straight in a chair, your back pressed against the back of it and your feet on the floor crossed at the ankles. Push up with the bottom leg and down with the other (actually, the ankles are pushing against each other). Hold for a count of 2, then release. Here you are forcing pressure at your ankles, which tightens the knees and also the thighs. Do 10, then switch the cross at the ankles.

This should take 30 seconds.

Repetitions: 10 each position

EXERCISE #2

Lie down on the floor or a mat with your feet flat against a wall, your legs at a 45-degree angle. Try to make your kneecaps come toward you (you'll be tightening your thighs as well). Do 25 of these. (See photo on page 91.)

This should take 30 seconds.

Repetitions: 25

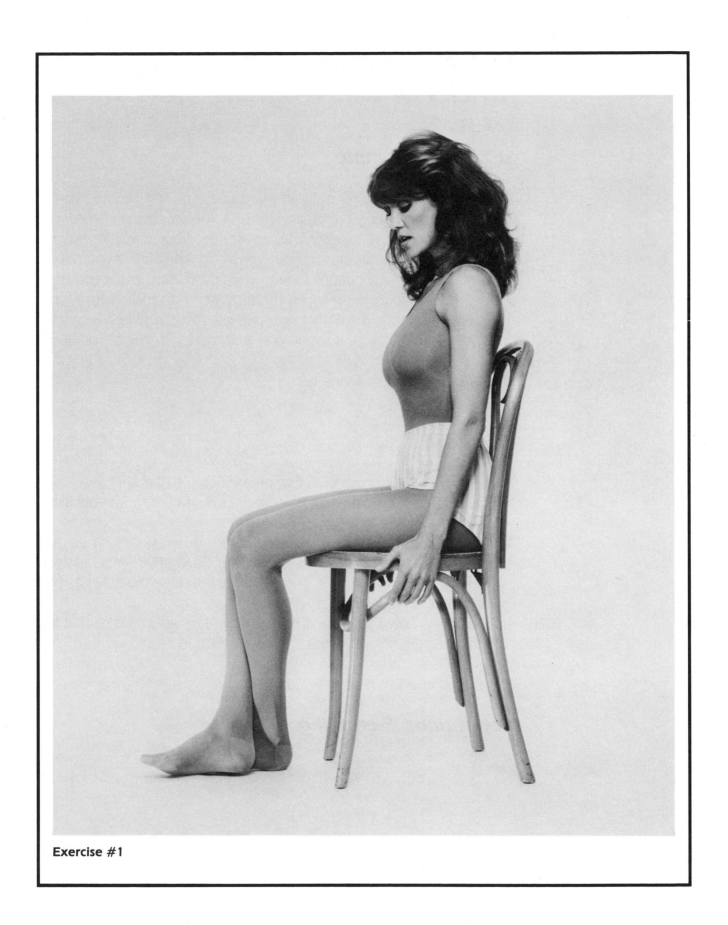

Exercise #1

SET X—Hamstrings (Backs of the Thighs)

SET TIME: 1 minute

The hamstrings are the tendons attached to the muscles in the back of the thighs (where you get a "charley horse"). They need some loosening up in most people. The idea is that if you keep your stomach muscles tight and your hamstrings loose, you won't hurt your back. If you have a weak abdomen, it will put pressure·on your lower back; and if you have tight hamstrings, your pelvis locks. The trick then is to make your whole body move in sync, to learn how to coordinate movement between your pelvis and your back so that when one area moves, so will the other.

WHERE: On a mat or on the bed.

EXERCISE

1. Lie down on your back on a mat on the floor or a bed.
2. Bring one leg toward your chest, knee bent, with arms at your sides and toes pointed.
3. Raise the straight leg as high as you can. When you can't go any farther, raise it another ½ inch, then lower slowly. Remember to keep your back against the floor. The tendency is to raise the pelvis as you raise your leg—don't do it!
4. Eventually, after some practice, you should be able to raise that leg straight up in the air. Do this 5 times for each leg.

This should take 1 minute.

Repetitions: 5 each leg

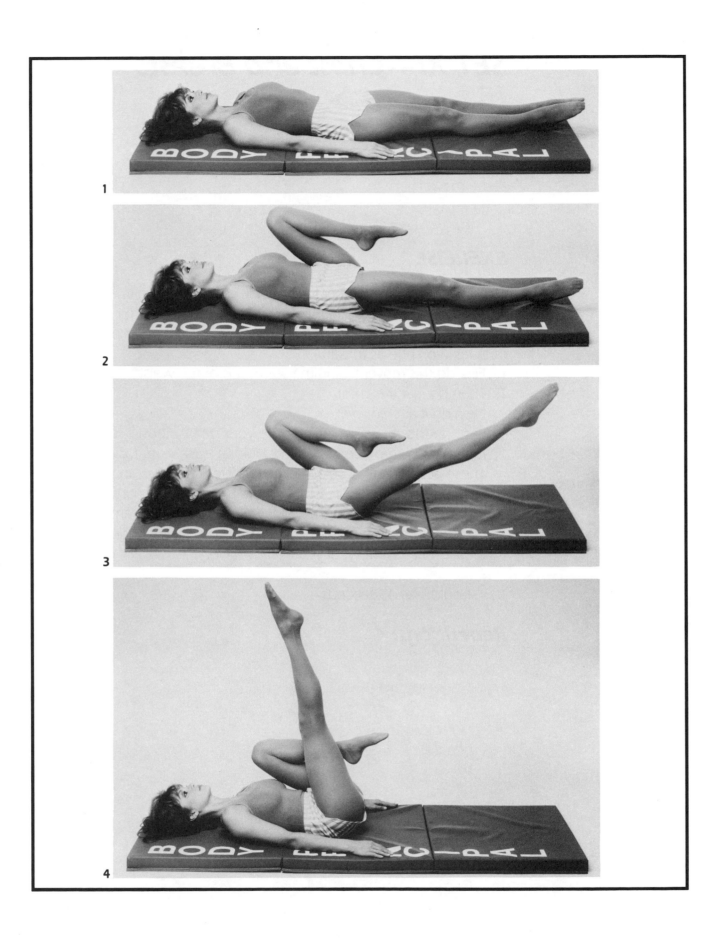

1

2

3

4

SET XI—Chest and Breasts

SET TIME: 45 seconds

WHERE: At home or in the office—anywhere but while waiting in line at the market.

EXERCISE

Clasp your hands together in front of you and push them together, pressing for resistance. Hold for as long as you can; try for a count of 4 (not too long or you'll get tired and the resistance that builds up the muscles won't be as forceful).

1. First do this movement with your hands at the waist.
2. Then do it at the chest.
3. Next do it at chin level.
4. Last, do this movement just above your head, elbows still bent, then repeat each step coming down. Hold at each level for a count of 4. These actions will develop several different muscles, including those in the arms and the breast. Keep the movement continuous—at the waist, at the chest and then higher. Repeat 4 times, remembering to breathe normally. Also remember: This is not meant to develop bigger breasts but to firm what you already have.

This should take 45 seconds.

Repetitions: 4

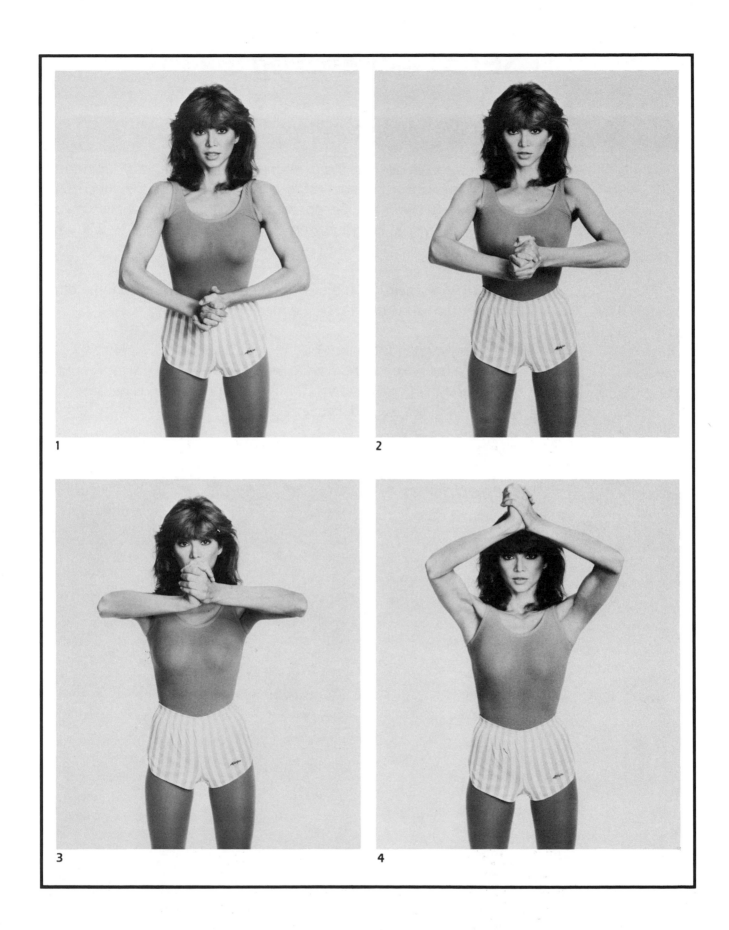

1

2

3

4

SET XII—Breathing

SET TIME: Approximately 45 seconds

This simple exercise firms the chest muscles and expands your lungs. It is great for your respiration—something we don't spend much time thinking about. But if you are not breathing properly (this applies in your daily life as well as for your exercise routines), nothing else will work properly either.

WHERE: Anywhere, any time. It can be done separately from the other exercises. You don't have to be warmed up for this one.

1. Clasp your hands behind you.
2. Take a deep breath and hold for as long as you can (try to a count of 10) and then let out slowly. This is great for your lungs because your chest muscles expand. Repeat 4 times.

This should take about 45 seconds.

Repetitions: 4

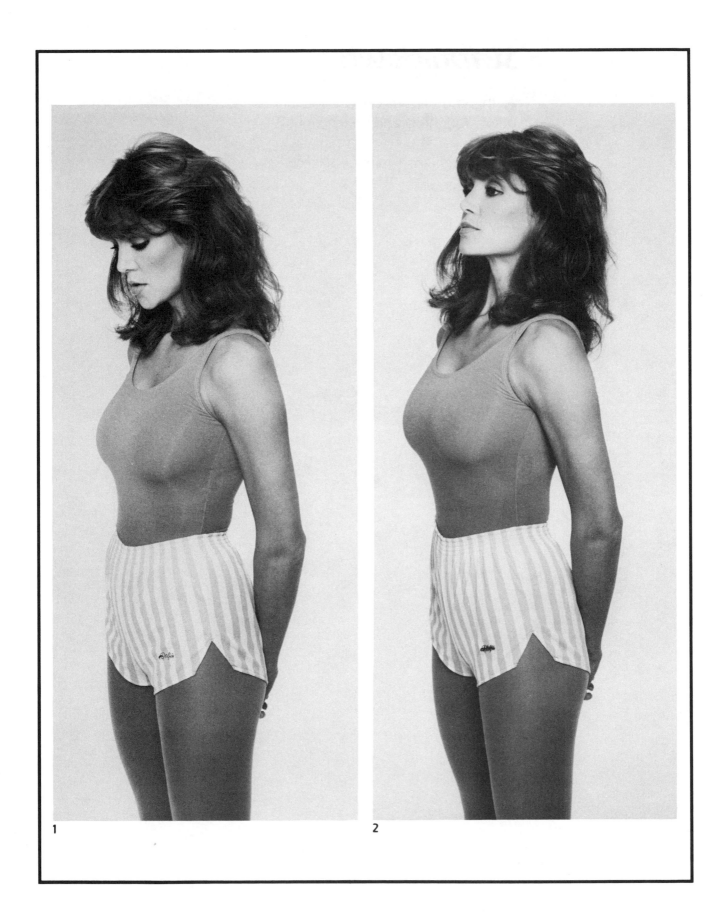

1   2

Warm-down

At the end of your exercise routine, do Warm-ups #2 and #3 to cool down your body and stretch it out.

This should take 1 minute, 30 seconds.

Warm-up #2

Warm-up #3

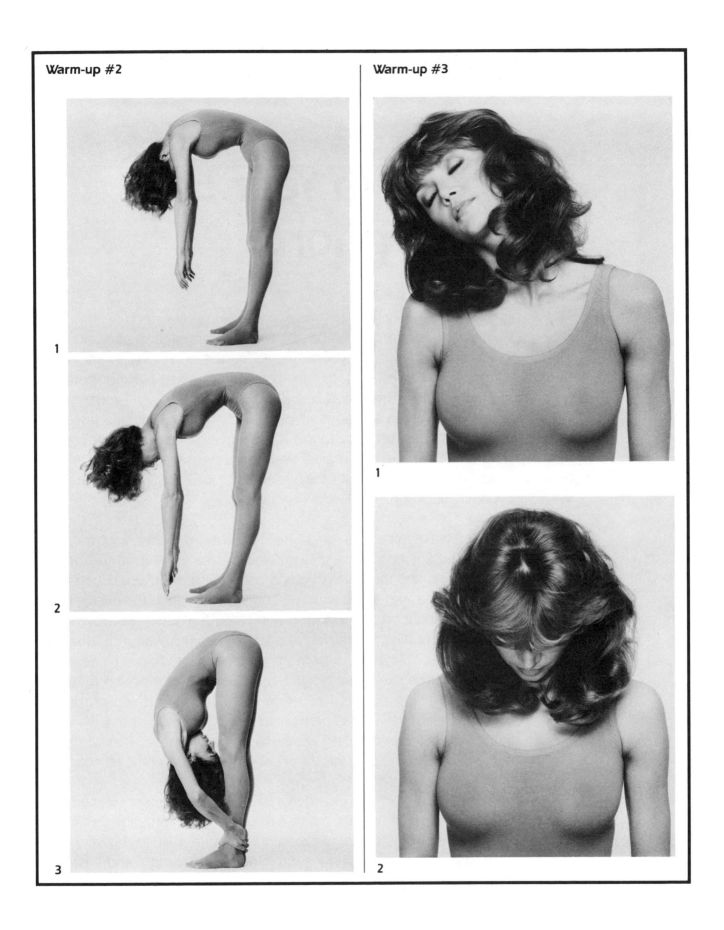

1

2

3

1

2

109

CHAPTER 4

Sports in Your Life: The Options

As far back as I can remember, I have been an eager participant in all kinds of sports. Years before I started the casual, occasional exercises that eventually became The Body Principal Program, I was playing sports. My mother, Ree, tells me I was somewhat of a tomboy. All I remember is that if you wanted someone to play Sunday touch football, basketball, baseball; if you needed a fourth for tennis; or if you just happened to have a boat and an extra pair of water skis, I was ready. I swam at the Y or at the swimming club; I rode horses at the local stables; I rode my bike everywhere. If anyone called—I was ready.

I did it because it was fun.

Sure, it was competitive—and I loved the challenge. Sure, it was social—and I loved the friendships, the camaraderie, the team spirit, the encouraging cheers and the understanding pats on the shoulder. When I was young my dad was in the air force, and we moved around every year or so. For me sports were a way of making friends in each new town.

But, most of all, participating in a sport, particularly an individual one like running or bicycling or swimming, gave me a chance to be active, to do something with my body. I could let it all out—push myself as hard as possible—do fifty laps or ski till my knees buckled or run till I was sure even the wind couldn't catch me. Or I could ease up—slither in the water, letting my mind wander and my body relax. I could sit back in the saddle, riding through the silent woods, taking time to notice the things around me I so often forgot.

As I grew older, my life changed. I traveled, built a career, worked hard, changed roads, came back again. I matured and eventually settled into a life that is happy, routine yet exciting. Through it all, to this very day, I have kept up my tennis, my swimming, my running—and I can still throw an occasional block.

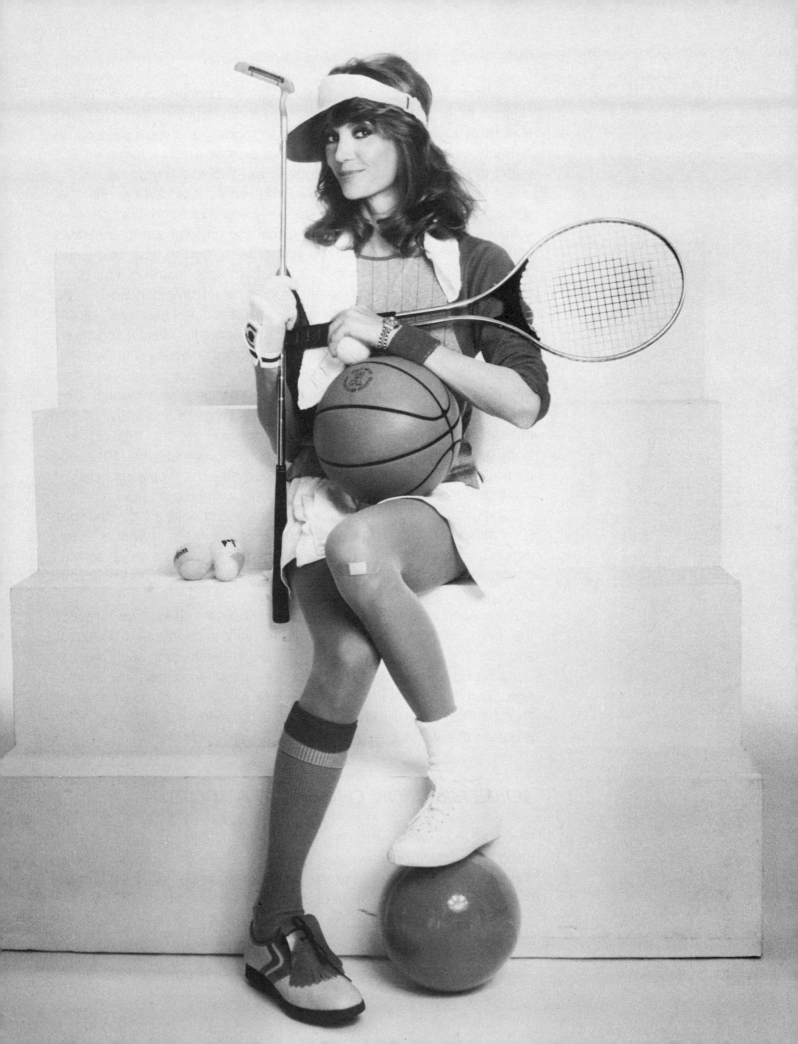

I believe that participating in sports is a good optional addition to our exercise program. But if you simply hate sports activities, forget it. Don't read this chapter. Do The Body Principal Program, and you'll develop an enviable, strong body; or do the optional exercise machine program. But forget the sports—sports are something you should enjoy doing.

But, if you do enjoy sports, and if you want the added benefits that participating in a sport can give your body and your mind, read on.

Sports offer many benefits. One is that the physical activity increases your cardiovascular workout. You get more oxygen to your body, and you give your heart the workout it needs to keep it strong. This is an excellent, beneficial addition to our program of resistive exercise.

A second benefit of participating in a sport is that it exercises parts of your body without you consciously thinking about it. Different sports use different muscles. For example, swimming tones and uses virtually every muscle in your body, while bicycling is superb exercise for your legs and thighs. Thus, when you know what parts of the body your favorite sport helps, you can add it to your Body Principal Program and know that at the same time you are having a great time, you are also helping your body get into and stay in shape. Or, if you've never really thought about participating in a sport, this may be a good time to try one, especially if you know that you can combine having fun with keeping fit.

Sports also give you a recreational choice. You choose a sport that suits your personality. You can engage in either a solitary, individual sport, which gives you a chance to be alone, or a sport that is a group activity, where you can communicate with people and also stretch and help your body.

Every sport exercises some part of the body. In this chapter I discuss the sports I engage in or believe you may want to choose as an optional addition to our basic exercise program. Listed before each sport are The Body Principal exercises to emphasize for additional conditioning for that sport. Remember that I am assuming you will be doing the basic Body Principal Program daily. I have marked any changes and additions in the exercises that will aid in preparation for playing each sport.

SOME HINTS ON CHOOSING A SPORT

There are two ways to choose a sport. One is to choose the one you are good at or have always wanted to try, just for the pleasure of doing it. You should know the parts of the body that sport will exercise, and do the Body Principal sets that strengthen the muscles it affects. If you have always wanted to swim, here you will find out what muscles swimming tightens and why I call it the "perfect" sport.

The other way to choose is to make note of the problem areas your body has (doing the program will make you acutely aware of each part of your body—so listing the areas you want to work on will be easy) and undertake a sport that works those muscles. An example: If you have a problem with your thighs, bicycling may be for you.

But remember, none of the sports will give you the isolated toning of the Body Principal exercises. Sports can strengthen and work a group of muscles but will not necessarily redefine nor resculpt your body the way you would like. These sports are to be done in addition to the daily Body Principal Program—by choice.

Before you make a decision, you may be interested in learning about the wide range of sports that women are involved in and succeeding in competitively these days. On both the professional and amateur levels, women are participating in swimming, riding, tennis, basketball, archery, volleyball, golf, bowling, skiing, soccer, bicycling, running, racquetball, squash, skating, roller-skating, diving, gymnastics, track—and many other sports.

BEGIN AT THE BEGINNING

Get some help.

I mean it. When you undertake a sport—any sport—get some assistance from a professional or at least advice from a friend who knows what he or she is doing. I would venture to say that none of you would consider driving a car without taking lessons first. How many of us would be able to make *salmon en croûte* or conduct Beethoven's Symphony no. 3 without at least a lesson or two? Well, neither should you undertake tennis or skiing or swimming or running without some help first. You will avoid making mistakes or picking up bad habits that will be harder to break later on. You will also lessen the possibility of injury. If you don't learn how to do a sport correctly, chances are you will end up working the wrong muscles, and that's neither worthwhile nor productive. The best lesson is this first one—ask someone who knows for help.

HOW OFTEN

As we have discussed, you can do The Body Principal Program of resistive exercises every day of your life. But participating in a sport is something else. Some sports you can engage in every day, but how many of us really have the inclination, energy or time? The last thing I want to do is make you feel the pressure of having to add yet another essential activity to your life. The Body Principal Program is easy to incorporate into your daily life, but sports are another matter. If you do take the option of adding one sport to your life style, you should try to do it at *least* once a week.

Most experts will tell you that it is better to engage in a sport every other day. Because you use the same muscles every time, you need to give them a day's rest (see the discussion on lactic acid and oxygen debt in Chapter 2). This is not true of resistive exercises because they do not work your muscles to the same degree. Some sports, like swimming, can be enjoyed every day because swimming works pretty much on the same principles as resistive exercises. Injury to a muscle is less of a problem, and you can always alternate swimming strokes so you work different muscles on consecutive days.

Make up your mind as to how often you can take part in your favorite sports activity. Don't force yourself, or you'll end up giving up rather quickly. Just as in The Body Principal Program, only do it as often as you realistically can, so you will take pleasure in it.

WEARING A BRA

I assume that for whatever sport you choose you will get the appropriate equipment. You won't play racquetball with a tennis racquet. You'll get the skis that are right for your height and skill level, and you'll wear running shoes that are comfortable, not just chic. But the most important item you should have is one you may not think about—a bra.

Any sport requires movement, and moving puts a strain on your muscles. Your chest muscles are particularly vulnerable in sports that involve movements such as running or jumping up and down. Thus, no matter what size breasts you have, I seriously advise that you wear at least a regular bra, if not a sports bra (you'll find the latter in department stores, lingerie shops and stores that sell athletic equipment). The bra you wear should limit the movement of your breasts (when you try one on, jump up and down to test it); it should be smooth so that it doesn't irritate your skin; and, if possible, it should be elasticized so it won't slip from its position.

WARM-UPS

As I emphasized when introducing my exercise program, it is very important for you to warm up (and cool down) before you engage in *any* sports activity. Many injuries occur because your muscles have not been stretched—they are too tight. A thorough warm-up can also prevent cramping.

The warm-up set in The Body Principal Program is a good one to do before and after most sports. Obviously, you don't need as extensive a warm-up before playing a round of golf as before running, but rather than trying to remember when you need to warm up and when you don't, make it a rule to *always* warm up and cool down when engaging in any sports activity.

Another hint—in some sports, such as swimming and running, it helps to slow down before you stop. This can be considered as part of the cool-down procedure.

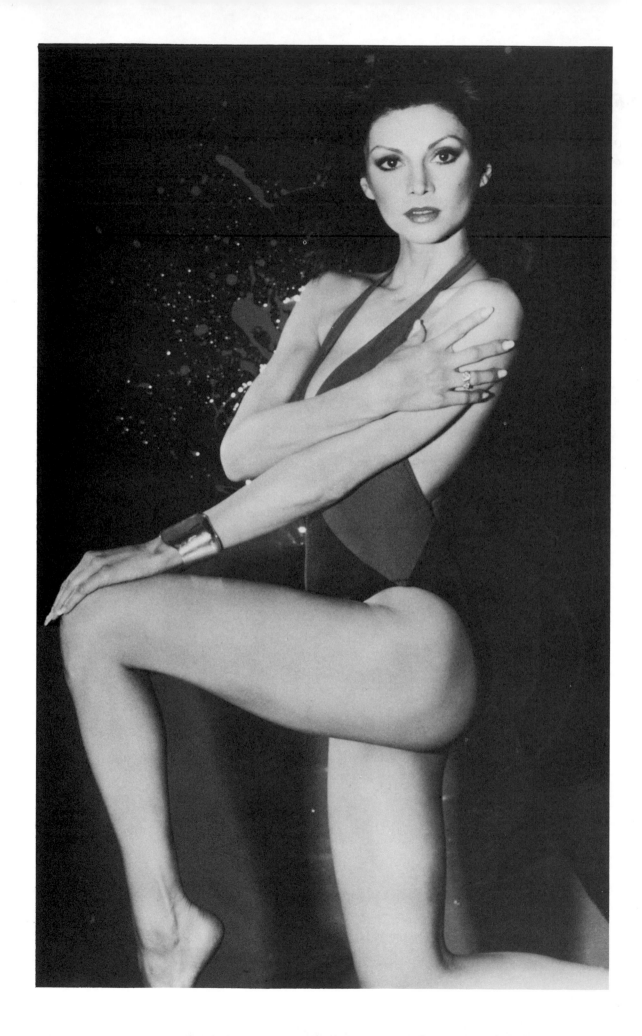

THE CHOICES

Swimming

THE BODY PRINCIPAL EXERCISES

Warm-ups
Set II—Arms and Shoulders; also do the optionals
Set IV—Stomach and Thighs; also do the optional
Set VII—Thighs: #1 and #2
Set VIII—Shoulders
Set XII—Breathing: Do for 1 minute

I am not alone in believing that my favorite sport, swimming, is also the "perfect" sport. Swimming works more muscles than any other sport, with the least chance of injury. The pull of gravity is diminished when you are in the water, and water acts as a natural resistor against which you work your muscles. In the water, you can use muscles you never knew you had. You elongate your spine without putting pressure on it because gravity is diminished; this makes swimming the perfect sport for those of us who have ever had any weakness in our backs. You extend, stretch and flex your arms, legs, neck, back, thighs, feet, shoulders, face, stomach—is there anything I missed?

The pool is a great place, not only to swim, but to do our resistive exercises. You can do the standing ones in the shallow end and the sitting ones on the steps of the pool.

Now this is not to say you can substitute swimming for a program of resistive exercises. Although swimming does make your muscles stretch and resist, it does not resculpt or finely define your muscles as well as The Body Principal Program exercises do.

With swimming, different strokes for different folks, as they say. I love to do the breast stroke with a flutter kick (rather than the frog motion that commonly accompanies it). I also like the side and back strokes. My chiropractor, Dr. Bruce Oppenheim, urges me to do the breast stroke on my back, because he believes it elongates the body, stretches it, and works the arm muscles. I also like to swim any stroke with my face in the water. It gives my facial muscles and my lungs and respiratory system a workout. No matter what stroke you prefer, you should elongate your stroke, stretching it out as much as possible. Swimming laps using just your arms or your legs is wonderful for those parts of your body.

Swimming, like many sports, provides an excellent release of tension. Being in the water is soothing and relaxing in itself, and a good workout will release built-up stress.

SOME ADDITIONAL HINTS: You should try not to swim in water that is too warm—over ninety degrees. Warm water makes you tired and is not conducive to exercising. Swim in water that is eighty degrees or cooler if you can.

Take advantage of water sports near your home. Swimming is not a sport reserved for those with private pools. There are public pools, YMCAs, health clubs, lakes, rivers, streams and oceans just waiting to be used.

Swimming is a flexible kind of sport because you can do it alone or with friends. I love to entertain friends in the pool—I have been known to bring out my water volleyball net and set up a game at the slightest urging. It's a wonderful way to enjoy the company of friends and exercise simultaneously. But when you feel the need, swimming is also *the* solitary sport of all time. Immersed in the water, in the rhythm of your stroke, you can truly be alone. This doesn't necessarily mean swimming unsupervised alone in a pool—it just means staying by yourself versus swimming, or playing, with others. Even in a public pool full of people you can find your own private space to think and relax, simply by swimming laps.

There have been times in my life when it has been difficult to find time to be alone. When I am away from home, working for months at a time, I often find a local Y or health club where, early in the morning or late at night, I can swim in quiet, in peace. There is a serenity about the water that I find enticing and soothing.

All this—and tight thighs, too.

Tennis and Racquetball

THE BODY PRINCIPAL EXERCISES

Warm-up: Do the running for 4 minutes
**Set II—Arms and Shoulders: #1, do 25; do optionals #1
and #2 (only 5 on each side)**
Set III—Calves and Ankles: #1
**Set IV—Stomach and Thighs: Do set twice and add the
optional**
Set XII—Breathing: Do for 1 minute

There have been hundreds of books written about tennis—entire books about tennis elbow, the back stroke, inner tennis, serving, and so on. My purpose here is simply to tell you what tennis does for your body, so that if it is the sport of your choice, you will know what it is doing to your muscles while you play.

First, lessons are a must. I have been playing tennis off and on for years, and I cannot imagine trying to play tennis for the first time without some sort of instruction. It is a game where every movement should be done correctly—or you will play badly, acquire bad habits that will be hard to get rid of and use the wrong muscles, which may result in injury. Many doctors say that most tennis injuries occur due to incorrect movements.

Tennis qualifies as a cardiovascular exercise; your heart rate will increase and your body will get a good workout. Tennis keeps you moving, of course, and you run more in singles than in doubles. It uses many muscles: You do extensions, tighten your legs, tone your thighs, and stretch your neck. It is also very good for muscle coordination.

There is a lot of lateral movement in tennis. You move your body sideways, across the court, rather than bending and moving up and down. Thus, there is little strain on the spine—except for serving overhead. Tennis builds up your endurance, makes your muscles stronger and gives your body a hard workout.

Tennis is a great way to release stress. Oh, my—how many times have I hit the ball pretending it was . . . well, never mind. Suffice it to say that the tennis court is a great place to get rid of your aggressions—much better than on the freeway. If you have to hit something, make it that ball, and take pride in the satisfaction of making it sail across the net and not return.

Tennis is excellent for working the muscles in your arms. When you serve, you work your shoulder and entire arm, and extend your whole body. When you stroke a strong forehand or a firm backhand, you build up your arm muscles. If you have had any problems with your arm muscles—particularly your elbow—try playing with a wooden-frame racquet. Some experts say it absorbs shock better than a metal one.

Many of the principles that apply to tennis also apply to racquetball, which has become a popular sport in recent years. Racquetball is faster than tennis. If you don't have quick reflexes and excellent depth perception, you may want to reconsider tennis.

Racquetball is easy to learn. The movements are less precise than in tennis; the racquet is smaller, shorter and easier to handle; and many who play both sports say it is easier to hit a racquetball. If you take up racquetball, you'll find that you give your body an excellent cardiovascular workout; but you will also get tired faster than you will playing tennis.

Racquetball will strengthen your thigh and calf muscles, and tighten your arm muscles. Doing The Body Principal Program's sets for the stomach (and thighs) and calves and arms will better prepare you for racquetball; and racquetball will in turn strengthen those muscles.

Racquetball, tennis, badminton, squash—all racquet sports are sports that women can enjoy, compete in comfortably, and use to build up our bodies. They are all relatively easy to learn and fun whatever your level of skill; and thus they may entice people who are not inclined to participate in sports. They build up your cardiovascular system. The equipment is relatively inexpensive and easy to find. There are courts everywhere: public outdoor courts in most towns and cities, indoor courts in high school and college gyms, and a variety of facilities at health clubs, public and private. You can start these sports at almost any age, as long as you have been exercising so that your body is strong and fit.

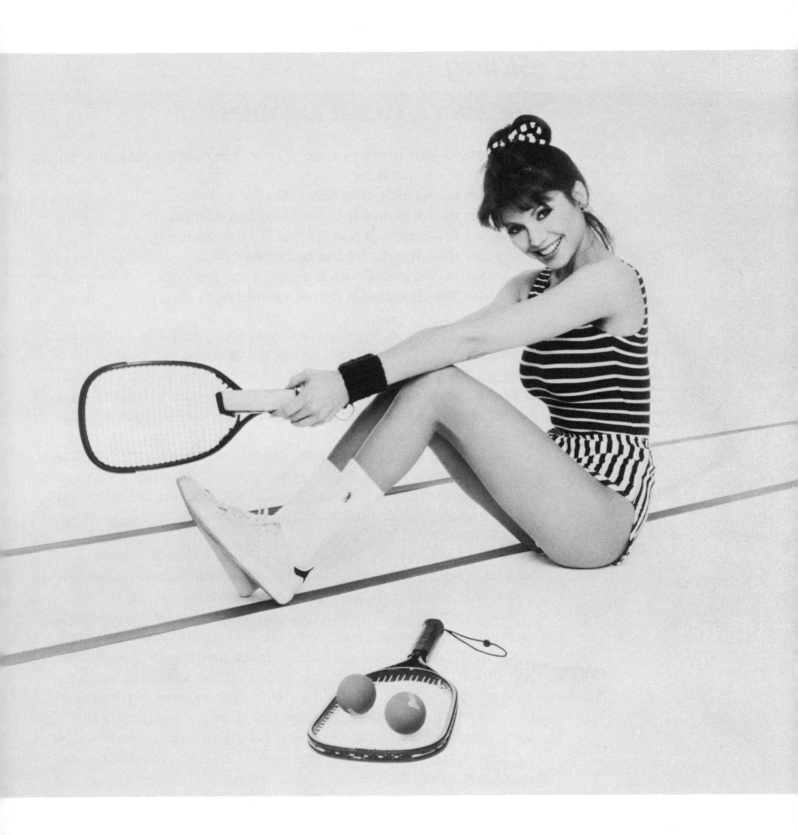

Skiing

THE BODY PRINCIPAL EXERCISES

Warm-ups: Don't run; do #2 for 2 minutes, optional for 1 minute

Set I—Buttocks and Pelvis: Do for 1 minute

Set II—Arms and Shoulders: Do the optionals

Set IV—Stomach and Thighs: Do the optional

Set VII—Thighs: Do the optionals

Set IX—Knees: Do each exercise for 1 minute

Set XII—Breathing: Do for 1 minute

Ever since I hurt my knee in Hawaii playing football, I haven't been able to take up skiing. I had to give up water-skiing, an old love of mine, both because of my knees and because it is just not easy to find a place to water-ski. The ocean may be just around the corner for those of us who live on either coast, but really, isn't it easier to pick up a racquet or jump in a pool?

I have always loved a snow-skiing excursion—the brisk, biting air; the glistening snow and awe-inspiring mountains; the shush of the skis as you round a curve or negotiate a mogul. There's the energizing feeling of the muscles in your body making you move—oh, what the heck, I think I'll unpack the skis.

Before taking up skiing, promise me you'll take lessons. And make sure your equipment is in good condition, because so much of skiing depends on it—working bindings, waxed skis, tight boots.

You really have to be in good physical condition to ski well without injuring yourself. First, you *must* warm up. Do the entire warm-up routine in the morning when you wake up. To make sure you are really flexible you should take an extra two minutes to do the stretching exercises. (Don't run—the air is thin in the mountains and running is neither necessary nor beneficial.) Do the entire Body Principal Program, including some optionals (see above) before you get on the slopes—and include the breathing exercise. In high altitudes it is particularly good to expand your lungs, slowly and easily.

Skiing is fantastic for your thighs; it really tightens them up. It is also good for your hips and your waist since there is a lot of rotation movement. In general it is an excellent sport for the lower half of your body and will give you superb control there, if you ski correctly (and this is where the lessons come in).

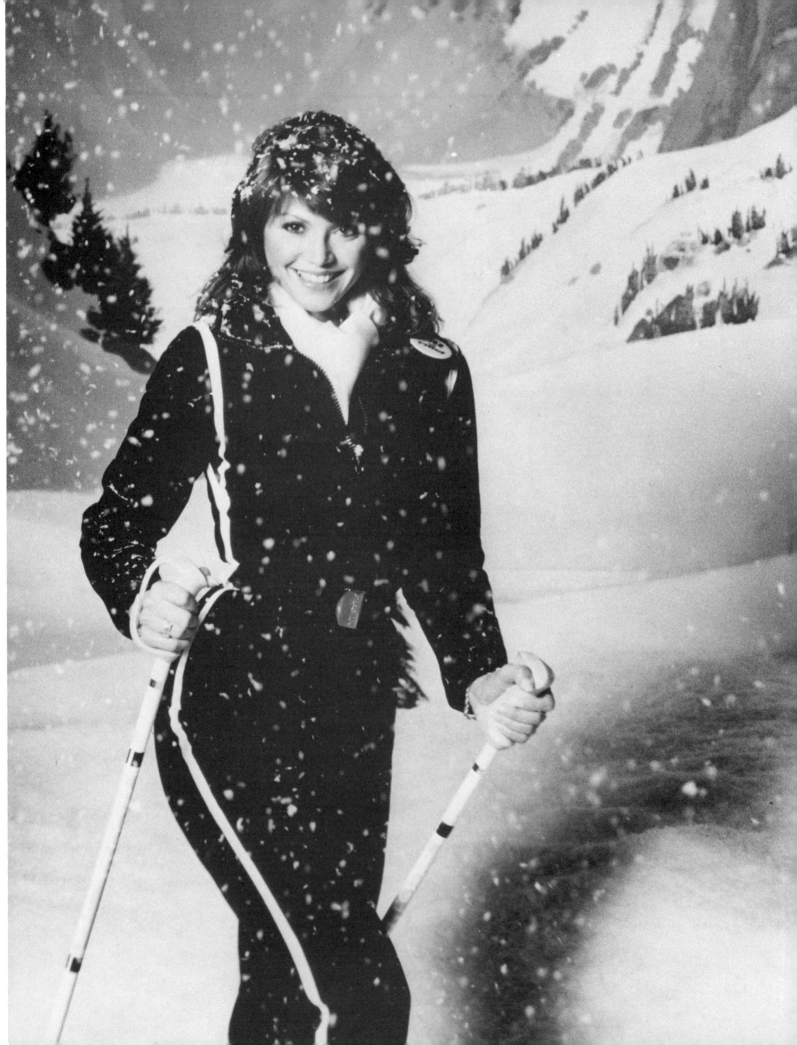

Cross-country skiing is good for your endurance. It is a hard workout that is excellent for your cardiovascular system, legs, calves, knees, waist, arms and hips.

Both types of skiing are good for your knees (if they haven't been damaged, like mine). The knee is a weak joint, only as strong as the muscles around it. If you've been doing The Body Principal Program and building up those knees and the muscles around them, you will greatly minimize knee injuries and be able to enjoy skiing without the fear of getting hurt.

Bicycling

THE BODY PRINCIPAL EXERCISES

Warm-up: Double up on #2
Set IV—Stomach and Thighs: Do the optional
Set VII—Thighs: Do the optionals
Set IX—Knees: Do for 1 minute each
Set X—Hamstrings: Do 10 times for each leg

If you know what these terms mean—drafting, hammering, honking, lead out, pull-off, spinning, breakaway—you are a serious cyclist, so skip this section and go on to golf.

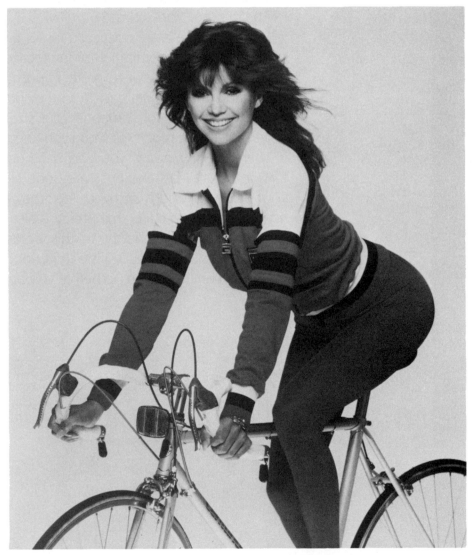

Recreational bicycling, popular in Europe for many years, has again become the rage in this country (it had a boom in the late 1890s—in 1895, Frankie Nelson won a six-day women's race in New York). Today it is increasingly popular all over the world, particularly for women. In fact women's cycling is included in the 1984 Olympics in Los Angeles.

Anyone can bike. (We're not talking about a stationary bike that you can ride in front of your television set watching the "Today" show—that's great exercise but it doesn't qualify as a sport.) Its relative ease and accessibility make bicycling an appealing sport. It is a quiet activity, one that even the shyest, most private people can do. Because it is easy, it also can boost the self-confidence of any reluctant sportswoman, or man. Many of those who try it become devotees overnight. If you don't like the water, the next best individual sport to take up is bicycling.

I love it. I ride my bike up and down the hills near my house as often as I can. (I have become very good at honking at unsympathetic motorists before they honk at me.)

Here are some basic practical rules for bicycling: Wear reflectors on the bike and on your clothing; wear protective headgear; follow traffic laws at all times; wear a hat to protect your face from the sun; don't wear long pants that can get caught in the spokes of the wheels; make sure your bike is made for someone your size; raise your handlebars if you have lower-back problems (you won't bend over as much).

There are few ways you can get hurt bicycling—unless it is by a foreign object (cars and trees are good examples). Bicycling is great for your legs, your thighs and your feet; they all get a good workout. If you ride for more than fifteen minutes, it is also good for your heart. Try going up a hill every now and then—this works your muscles and your heart harder. Like skiing, bicycling is a lower-body sport.

And remember, warm up before you begin.

Golf

THE BODY PRINCIPAL EXERCISES

Warm-ups
Set IV—Stomach and Thighs: Do the optional

Playing golf will give you more exercise than changing the channels on your television set, and I suppose it is better than not participating in any sport. It gets you out in the fresh air and makes you walk (carts are absolutely forbidden). But that's about it. Even the pros will tell you that

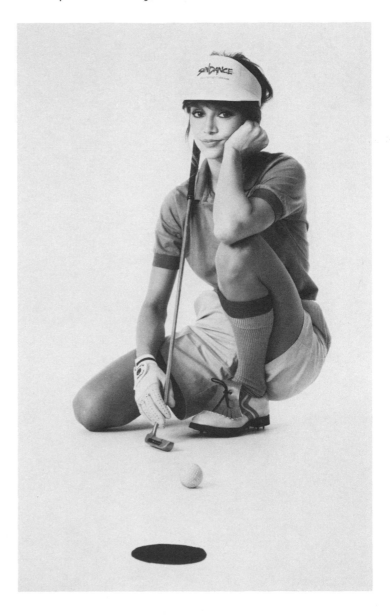

although golf takes a tremendous amount of skill, it is not a sport that gives the body a lot of exercise. It really is a relaxation sport—great for those of you who need a calm, nontaxing form of recreation that is slow and deliberate.

Golf does not tone any muscles. You do use your arms but not strenuously. You stand on your feet a lot, so if your back tends to get tired, you should strengthen your stomach muscles with the exercises I recommend for them (remember, a tight stomach takes the pressure off your back). But the sport itself does not give you muscle tone.

Now don't get me wrong. I like golf. And it does help you to develop superb concentration, timing, control and the ability to handle pressure. But it is not a cardiovascular nor a muscle-building sport. If you enjoy it, do it, but at least walk the course.

Bowling

THE BODY PRINCIPAL EXERCISES

Warm-ups
Set II—Arms and Shoulders: Do the optionals
Set IX—Knees: Do each exercise for 1 minute

I bowl—not well, but I enjoy it. It's fun and gives me a chance to spend time with friends. I have never really thought about bowling as a sport that develops your muscles—mostly because people bowl once, maybe twice, a week, which is not enough to give your body a true workout.

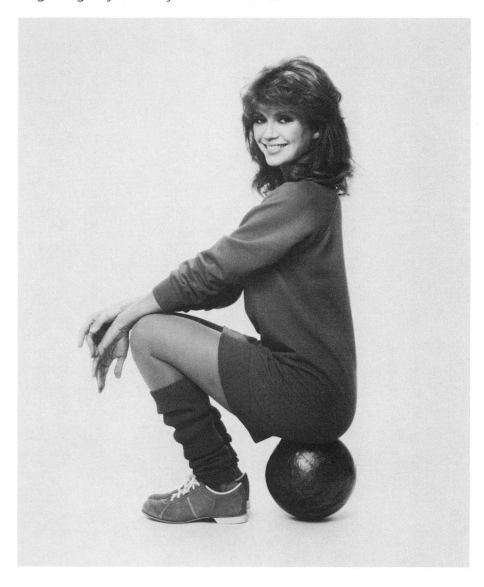

There are some things you should be aware of if you are a bowler. Bowling is not a cardiovascular sport; it is relaxing, a social sport that requires skill but not necessarily great strength or mobility.

Before bowling, it is important to do our warm-up set for stretching and flexing. Most people don't think it is necessary, but professional bowlers do it—so why not you? You should also note that when people hurt themselves bowling it is usually when they pick up the ball. Many people bend over and, forgetting to bend their knees, they pick up the heavy ball and pull the muscles in their backs. So take care—remember to *always* bend your knees.

It helps to have strong arms in bowling, just for that forward throwing motion of the ball. If you bowl often enough, you may build up your arm muscles; and vice versa, if you concentrate on the arm exercises in The Body Principal Program, it will be easier for you to bowl.

Running

THE BODY PRINCIPAL EXERCISES

Warm-ups
Set III—Calves and Ankles: #1, be sure to do 50; do #2; do
#3
Set IV—Stomach and Thighs: Do the optional
Set VII—Thighs: Do optionals
Set XII—Breathing: Do for 1 minute

There have been almost as many books written about running as all other exercises combined. Running and jogging have become prevalent all over the world. I can understand the passion—I have been running for the last three years. I know the energy it takes, the high it provides. Running keeps you in shape. It's the most popular cardiovascular exercise there is. And for me it's one of the best ways to release built-up tension and stress.

Running is exhilarating—you're racing with the wind, oxygen is flowing to all parts of your body—you feel a burst of energy that makes you feel truly alive.

Running uses a lot of muscles (but not as many as swimming—and it's not as safe for your body). Obviously, you build up your legs. If done correctly running builds up your arms, too. You breathe deliberately while running, so you are expanding your lungs and giving your body a lot of oxygen. You burn up energy and thus may burn up unwanted calories.

However, there are a few things worth noting to avoid trouble. One is that running pounds your spine, knees and worst of all, your feet—particularly if you run on concrete. I see people running up and down the streets and I just cringe. If you want to build up your leg muscles, do it on soft ground, on dirt. Run in the park, on the school track, on the beach (now that's hard!)—but not down Main Street.

Be aware of motorists. They are not always watching for you, and there are far too many accidents involving cars and runners. Wear bright colors, and, if you must run at night, wear reflectors all over your body. They could very well save your life. Remember, you are defeating the whole purpose of keeping in shape if you get hit by a car.

Wear a bra when you run. It's a must. Even with a bra you may feel some soreness in your breasts, so try running with your hands crossed over your breasts. (I have found that it relieves temporary pain in the chest muscles.)

Some women complain that running increases their urinary frequency. Doing pelvic exercises to tighten the PC muscle (see Chapter 3, Set II—Buttocks and Pelvis, and Chapter 7, the section on Sex and Exercise) will help. The Body Principal pelvic exercise is one that doctors recommend for women for whom urinary frequency is a common problem. And it helps fast!

If you tend to have back problems, try *walking fast.* Walking at a brisk rate increases your heart workout without risk of injury to your back. Walking doesn't jar your skeletal system as running does. Actually, I think that walking at a fast pace (this really is not strolling, folks—I mean walking very, very fast) has all the advantages of running and none of the disadvantages.

If you want to see the difference that running or walking fast make in your cardiovascular system, try this. Before and within five seconds after running or walking fast, check your pulse to measure the exact rise in your heart rate. To find your pulse, place your fingertips on the inside of your wrist, or on your neck, just below the angle of your jawbone. Count the number of beats in a six-second period; add zero to that number and you will have your heart rate. If your normal heart rate is between 60 and 90 beats per minute, and you find that right after running your rate increases to 130 or 160 per minute, you have given your body a good cardiovascular workout. Doctors also say that if your pulse drops 30 to 40 beats in the first minute after you have finished running or other exercise, you are probably in good physical shape.

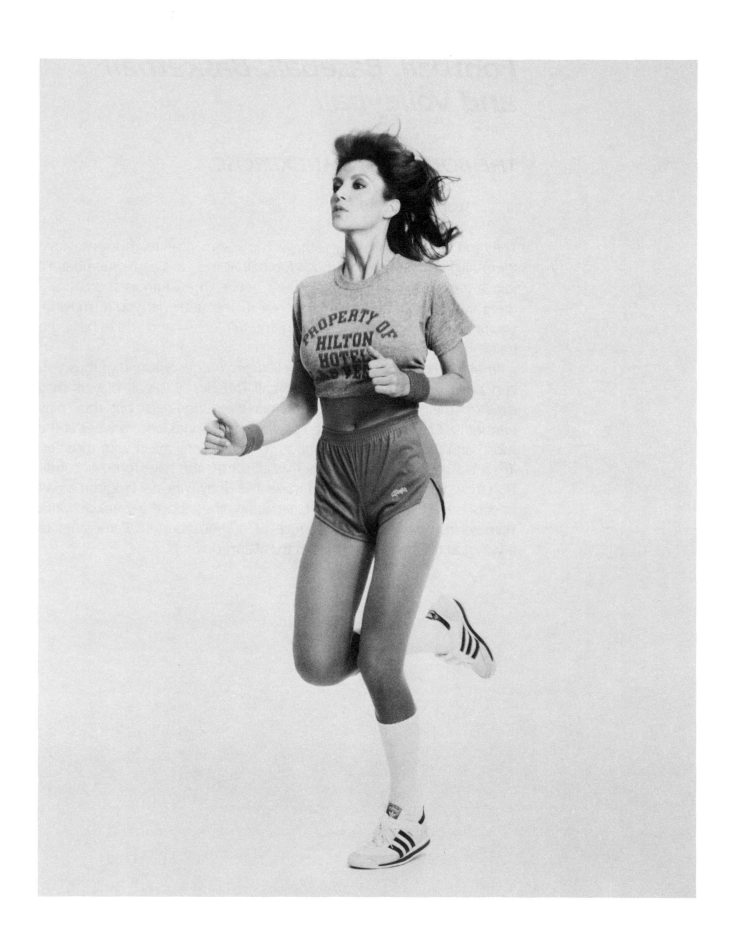

Football, Baseball, Basketball and Volleyball

THE BODY PRINCIPAL EXERCISE

Warm-ups: Always

They sort of go together, don't they? The all-American team sports. I love them all! I've been playing touch football as long as I can remember. I'll join a basketball game at a minute's notice. These group sports are a great way to get exercise. You're out in the fresh air, you're moving, you're running, your circulation is going full force—and you're having a ball.

In all of these sports, the basic exercise you get is running; thus you can build up your leg, thigh and calf muscles. Baseball players may develop their arm muscles and work their shoulders, but they play frequently. Chances are you'll be playing these sports once a week at the most, and that is really not enough to significantly affect your muscles. There's a danger in these once-a-week sports: You have to be in condition to avoid injuries. Once you make The Body Principal Program a part of your daily routine, you'll be able to join in these once-a-week activities with relative ease and less chance of hurting yourself. Remember to always do the stretch exercises in the Warm-ups.

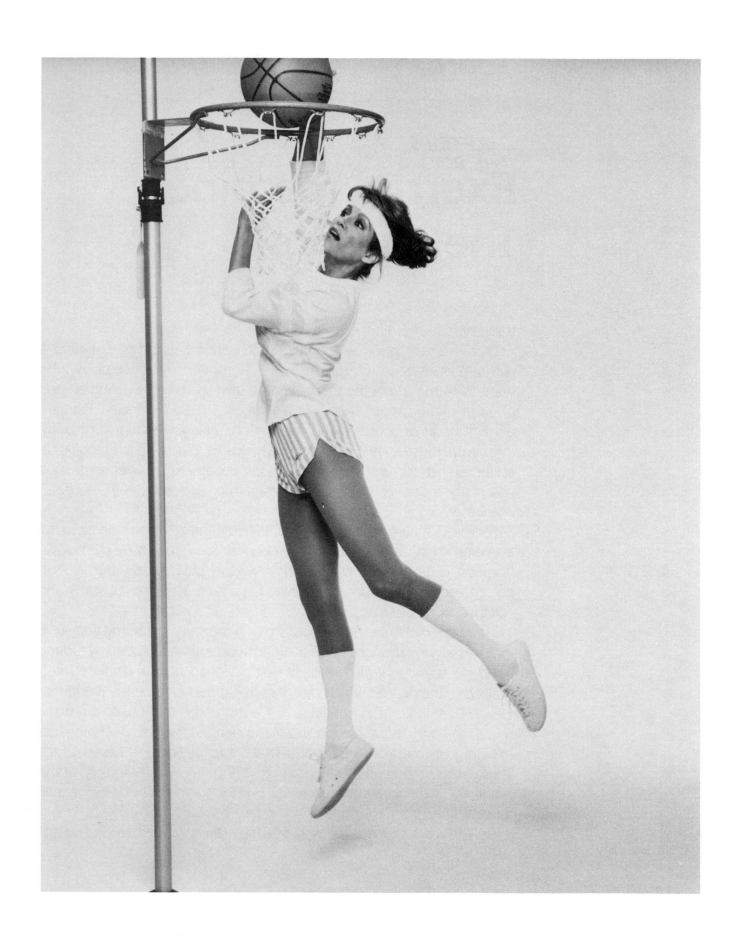

CHAPTER 5

Exercise Machines: The Options

Why exercise machines?

That is a very good question, and the answer is simple. Starting a program of exercise using machines is an option for those of us who want to further strengthen our muscles, give them more definition and give our cardiovascular systems a workout. If The Body Principal Program becomes part of your daily life, you will be able to resculpt your body, tone your muscles and get into great shape. But there are additional options for those who may want more: Becoming involved in a sport you enjoy is one; embarking on a program of exercising with machines is another.

For me, it started that day in Dallas when I agreed to participate in the television show called "Battle of the Network Stars." As I have mentioned, I agreed to do the show believing I was in great shape, but when I decided to practice running a mile, I made it a couple of yards and collapsed!

I still remember my shock and dismay at the sorry shape my body was in. I had always thought I was a strong woman—and suddenly I found I had no stamina at all. I realized that I needed help and immediately walked to the nearest health club, which happened to be the President's Health Club in Dallas. I explained to the instructors that I had committed myself to doing this television show and begged them to help me—not to win, just to make sure I would make it to the closing credits of the show. When I accepted the challenge, I had visions of winning; at this point my intention was simply to still end up standing. I was committed to changing my deplorable condition so I would not make a fool of myself in front of America. And this motivation proved to be half the battle.

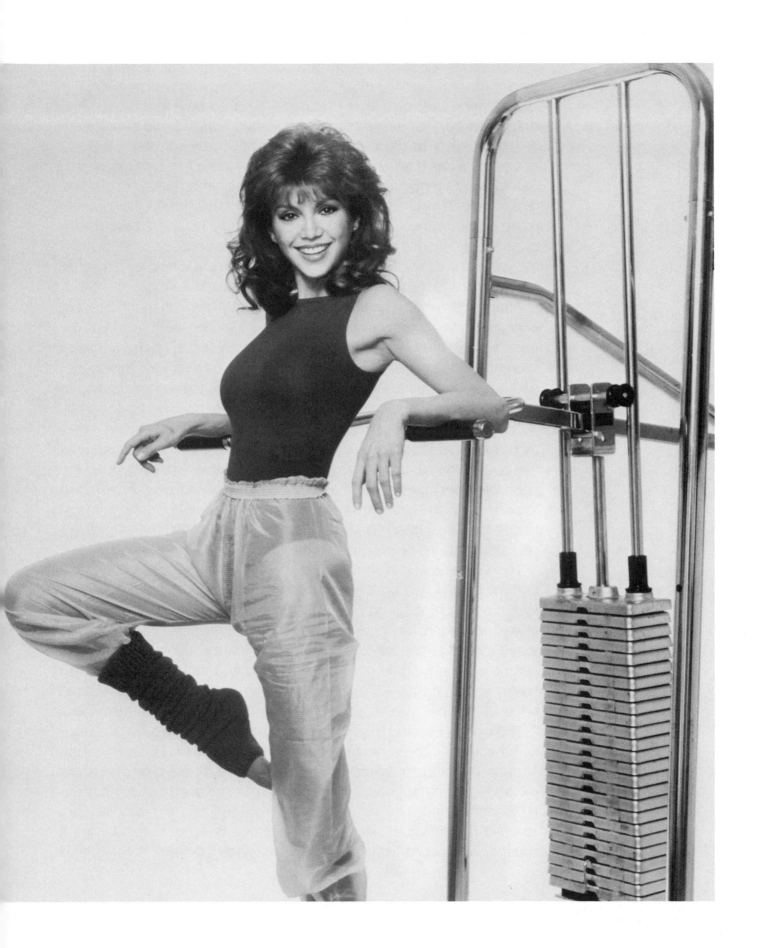

I realized that attitude is everything. Deciding that you are going to do something makes all the difference in your subsequent performance. The cliché "mind over matter" is overused—but I do believe it is true. And that's how I did it. I worked on the set filming "Dallas" all day, and then at night I went to the club and worked out (I think in three weeks I missed only one day). The instructors put together a program for me that would build up my strength, suggesting specific machines for my arms, legs, stomach, and so on. I worked hard. At times I thought I'd never make it, but my motivation was strong. Every time I pushed that bar with my arms, I knew that the next time it would be easier. Each time I pushed the weights with my legs, I knew that the next time it would be smoother. I was right, and the instructors were right. It worked.

After three weeks, I had tremendous strength and stamina. I felt more energetic and more vibrant. I didn't think I looked very different; the exercises I was doing were not designed to reshape my body but to strengthen it. But I noticed the change. When I moved, I felt a strength I had not had in years. I truly felt wonderful! There was a new feeling of accomplishment, of contact with and control over my own body.

The story had a happy ending—I went on the show and I won. Then, as suddenly as I had started, I stopped going to the club—stopped all exercises. When it came time to do another "Battle" show, I began the crash program again—and then stopped after it was over. It seems so foolish, now, this starting and stopping every time. I suppose it just hadn't sunk in; it hadn't occurred to me that I could feel this strong, this confident, this terrific every day of my life.

Then came that day in the kitchen, when Annie pointed out to me that my behind was on its way down—literally. That's when I found an incentive that was strong enough for me; it was personal and this time it was permanent. I decided to exercise for me, because I didn't like the way I looked or the way I felt. Not for the money. Not to avoid embarrassment in front of the public. Just for me. And for the last few years I have been doing my Body Principal Program, and occasionally—sometimes three times a week, sometimes once—I work out with machines.

The option of using machines is one that I love. It gives me a chance to have even more control over the condition and shape of my body. Though my program keeps me toned and tight all the time and keeps my body looking as good as it can look, I have the option of doing more. If I want to develop the muscles in my back, I use the machines. If I want to build my arms just a little more, I use free weights. When I want a tougher workout to get my cardiovascular system going, I choose circuit weight training with the machines. When I have some extra time in my hectic schedule, I go to the machines, and I exercise.

The exercises described here form a program that I use and really enjoy, put together by Dr. Paul Ward, Director of Education, Research, and Development for the Health and Tennis Corporation of America.* I know it is effective—it is the one that helps me. I recommend it as an option for those of you who want to extend your exercising beyond the basic Body Principal Program.

THE TRUTH ABOUT EXERCISE MACHINES

First, let's get rid of a couple of misconceptions about exercising with machines. Most women fear that using machines will give them massive muscles like a man. This is virtually impossible. The main factor in muscle growth is the amount of androgens (male hormones) manufactured in your system. Since the adrenal glands produce small amounts of androgens in women, such massive bulges occur only if there is a serious malfunction of these glands. So, relax; you can use machines without developing huge, masculine muscles.

Another common misconception is that muscles have to be large in order to be strong. This is simply not true. (Just ask the last person I hit in the stomach on a dare. He commented that such a small, thin woman like me could not hit hard. I couldn't resist the challenge, and I swear I didn't hurt him—not a lot.) Research has shown that women seem to increase their strength by improving their abilities to utilize the nervous system more effectively, not by drastically increasing their muscle mass.

There are as many theories of training with weight-loaded machines as there are people training with them. It is very difficult to separate the truth from the myth, but what we can do is to turn to common sense and science. Thus, the purpose of this section is to present some basic principles of scientific weight-training programs.

There are three basic principles that explain what happens when you use weights for physical training. They are:

1. A heavy amount of weight and few repetitions produce strength and size.

*Holiday Health Spas, Vic Tanny Health Clubs, President's Health Clubs, Chicago Health Clubs, Jack LaLanne Health Spas (New York)

2. A lighter amount of weight and more repetitions produce local muscle endurance and definition.

3. The two principles are not interchangeable. We can use different programs to produce different results, depending upon the objective.

The type of program I use when I want to gain more strength and greater visual definition in certain muscles is called circuit weight training (CWT). According to Dr. Ward, the term was devised by researchers at the University of Leeds in England in 1955. Since that time, CWT has been used primarily for training athletes and soldiers. In the early 1970s, Don Wildman introduced CWT as a means of popular physical training in the Chicago Health Clubs. Subsequently, Dr. Ward researched, organized and systematized CWT as an effective exercise program.

What is circuit weight training? According to Dr. Ward, it involves performing a series of exercises that conditions every major muscle group in a nonstop sequence, while alternating muscle groups for consecutive exercises. Thus, you might do an exercise for the thighs, followed by another exercise for the arms, and so on. Work periods are usually thirty seconds, alternating with rest periods of fifteen seconds (you exercise for thirty seconds without stopping, then rest for fifteen seconds and then go directly to another exercise). Each exercise conditions a different muscle group (much the way The Body Principal Program does). For general fitness (as an optional addition to The Body Principal Program), each exercise is repeated between twelve and fifteen times (beginners can do less or can put less weight on the machines).

Research has shown that CWT increases strength, local muscle endurance and cardiovascular endurance. It reduces orthopedic stress (pressure on the joints and bones of the body), while at the same time reducing body fat. The typical CWT program involves the following muscle groups:

Muscle Group	Machine/Exercise
Fronts of thighs	Knee Extension
Shoulders and arms	Shoulder Press
Backs of thighs	Leg Curl
Upper back and arms	Pull-down
Hips and legs	Leg Press
Chest/front, shoulders and arms	Chest Press
Waist	Rotary Torso Machine
Backs of arms	Push-down

Muscle Group	Machine/Exercise
Lower back/hips and legs	Hip-and-Back Machine
Abdominals	Abdominal Machine
Chest	Vertical Fly
Hip flexors/abdominals	High Chair

One of the benefits of CWT is the cardiovascular workout you will receive. As you are doing the exercises, you will be able to feel your heart pounding faster than it usually does. This is good! One of the benefits of using these machines is that your heart rate increases and is sustained throughout the program, producing a rate ranging from 130 to 160 beats per minute.

HINTS FOR EXERCISING WITH MACHINES

1. Warm up before you begin the exercise routine. Do the warm-up set from The Body Principal Program or run in place or use a stationary bike (most health clubs have them). Never exercise on the machines without warming up, thus stretching your muscles.

2. Remember to watch your breathing. Do not hold your breath while exercising. Exhale when pushing or pulling against the weight. When in doubt, just breathe normally.

3. As you are exercising on a machine, try to be aware of the muscles you are working. I have always believed that if you focus on what you are doing, if your mind and your body are in tune, the results will be better. So leave those thoughts of grocery lists and calls missed at home. Concentrate on exercising.

4. You may start with any exercise, although it is advisable to begin with the same exercise each time. This may be difficult at a club because the machine you would like to start with may be in use, but if you can, establish a routine order of exercises.

5. Work through your program according to your physical capability. Don't overdo it. Don't perform for others. Just do as much as you feel comfortable with. You don't have to prove anything to anyone—and if you overdo it, chances are you will injure yourself.

6. Don't overexert; your pulse should range between 130 and 160. If you feel short of breath, slow down and stop.

7. Do all the exercises without stopping. Continue the movement you are doing to the end. Move smoothly—jerking is not allowed.

8. Select a weight that is comfortable enough so that you can do twelve to fifteen repetitions, without stopping, in the suggested thirty-second intervals.
9. Your weight loads should ideally be increased regularly (about once every two weeks if you are going three times a week) for continuous progress. For a maintenance program, use the same moderate load every time.
10. Cool down, just as you warmed up. Walk, run, bike or do my stretch warm-up set again for about five to ten minutes.

Using machines as an optional addition to The Body Principal Program has many benefits. A program such as circuit weight training will increase your strength and local muscle endurance and reduce body fat. It is also not too inconvenient—one to three thirty-minute sessions a week is realistic even for the busiest woman. You can go more often if you have the time; it won't hurt because of the moderate intensity of circuit weight training.

When you are working with machines, you do so in an enjoyable, noncompetitive social atmosphere that can contribute to your persistence in and dedication to exercise. You don't have to perform in front of an exercise class led by a teacher encouraging you to do "still more," nor in front of a tennis partner bent on winning by running you ragged. There is no peer pressure egging you on to do more than you can or should. Just as The Body Principal Program is geared especially for you, so is a CWT program designed only for you to do as much and as well as you can.

Before you embark on the program that I use, remember two things. The first is to breathe properly throughout your exercises. I know that I have reminded you of this before, but you would be surprised to find out how many people forget to breathe. So breathe out when exerting pressure, and breathe in as you return to your starting position. If you aren't sure of what you should be doing, just breathe naturally. Above all—don't hold your breath while exercising.

The second is to know that the repetitions of each exercise depend on the condition of your body, how much weight you are lifting, and your goals for using these machines. At a health club, there will be an instructor to help design a program for you. Tell him or her your reasons for working with machines—your goals, your physical condition, your time availability and constraints, your own appraisal of your capabilities. I must emphasize that to get the most out of any program of exercise with machines and to minimize the risk of injury, you need expert advice. On these pages are illustrations and explanations of the exercises and machines that I use when I choose to add this type of exercise to my Body Principal Program. Study these, but be sure to also get invaluable individual instruction at your local health club.

Now, here we go.

Knee Extension

(BY UNIVERSAL)

PURPOSE: This exercise conditions the fronts of the thighs.
MUSCLES: Fronts of the thighs (the quadriceps)
TIME: Do for 30 seconds, as many as you can up to 15.

1. Sit on the machine with the fronts of your ankles under the pads.
2. Extend your knees until straight. Return to the starting position and repeat.
3. This exercise may be done with both legs at the same time or by alternating each leg. Work through the full motion. Don't stop or jerk; keep it smooth.

Repetitions: 15

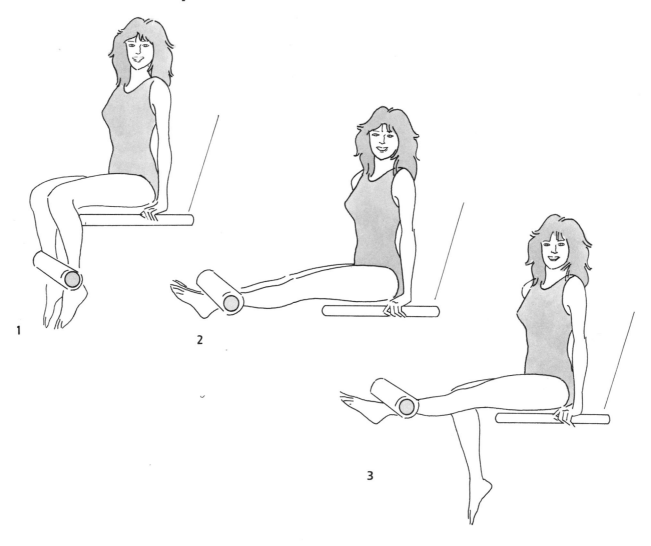

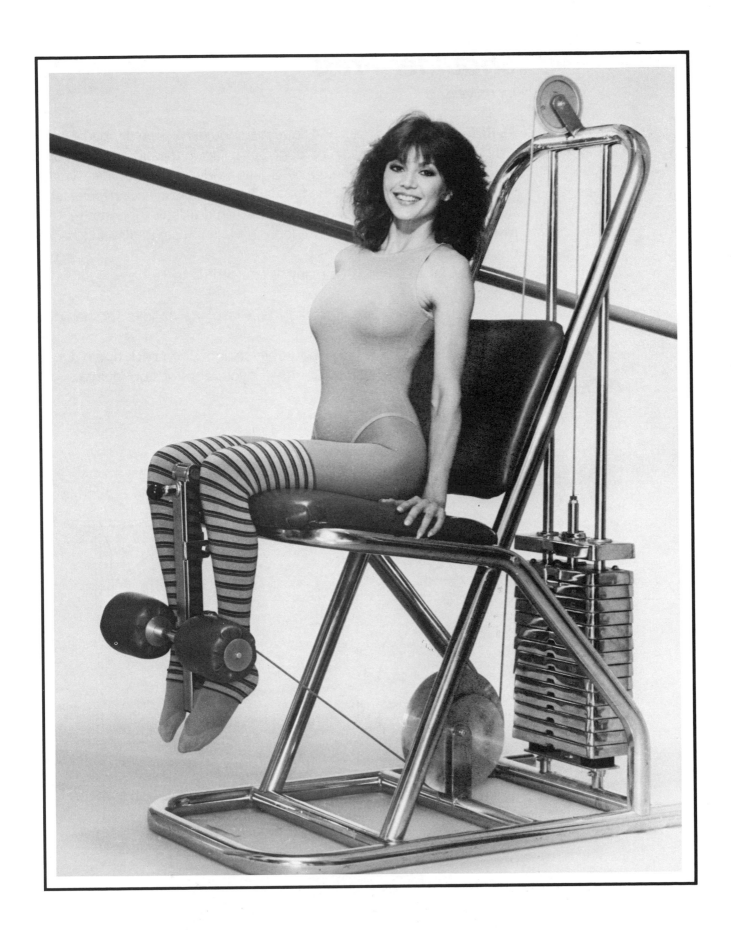

Shoulder Press

(BY UNIVERSAL)

PURPOSE: This exercise conditions the shoulders, shoulder girdle and the backs of the arms. It can be done either facing toward or away from the machine. The grip should be a little wider than shoulder width. Sitting on the stool protects the back by inhibiting low-back hyperextension. The feet can be either on the floor or on the chair supports.
MUSCLES: Shoulders (deltoids), upper back (shoulder girdle) and backs of the arms (triceps)
TIME: Do for 30 seconds, as many as you can up to 15.

1. Sit facing away from the machine. Grasp the handles at shoulder height with elbows bent.
2. Push arms up until your elbows are straight, then back down. Do it slowly, moving smoothly. Do not jerk your arms or stop midway.

Repetitions: 15

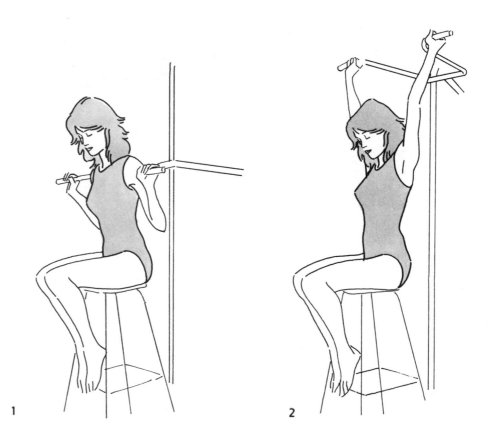

1

2

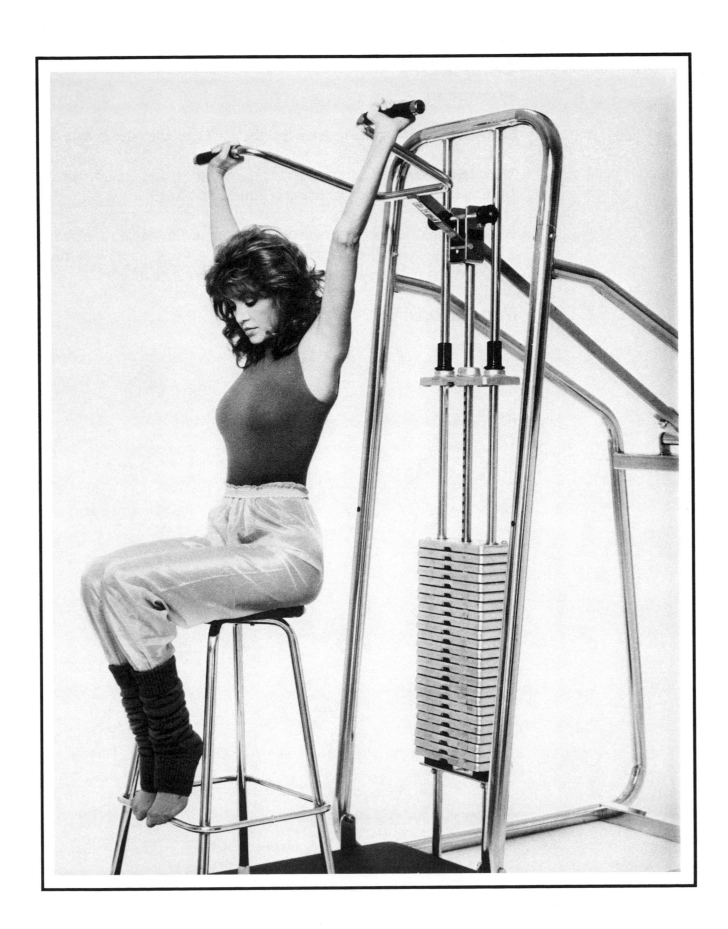

Leg Curl

(BY UNIVERSAL)

PURPOSE: This exercise conditions the backs of the thighs and the calves.

MUSCLES: Backs of the thighs (hamstrings) and the calves (gastrocnemii)

TIME: Do for 30 seconds, as many as you can up to 15.

1. Lie on your stomach with the backs of your ankles against the pads.
2. Bend your knees until they form a 90-degree angle, then bring them down again. Don't jerk the motion, and complete it fully.

Repetitions: 15

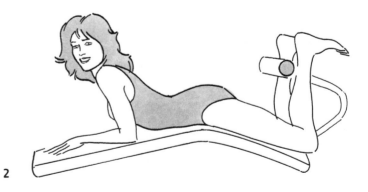

1

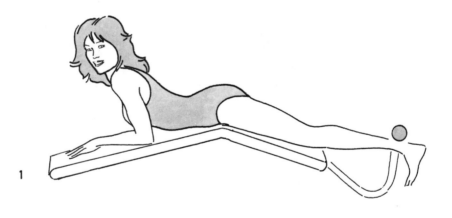

2

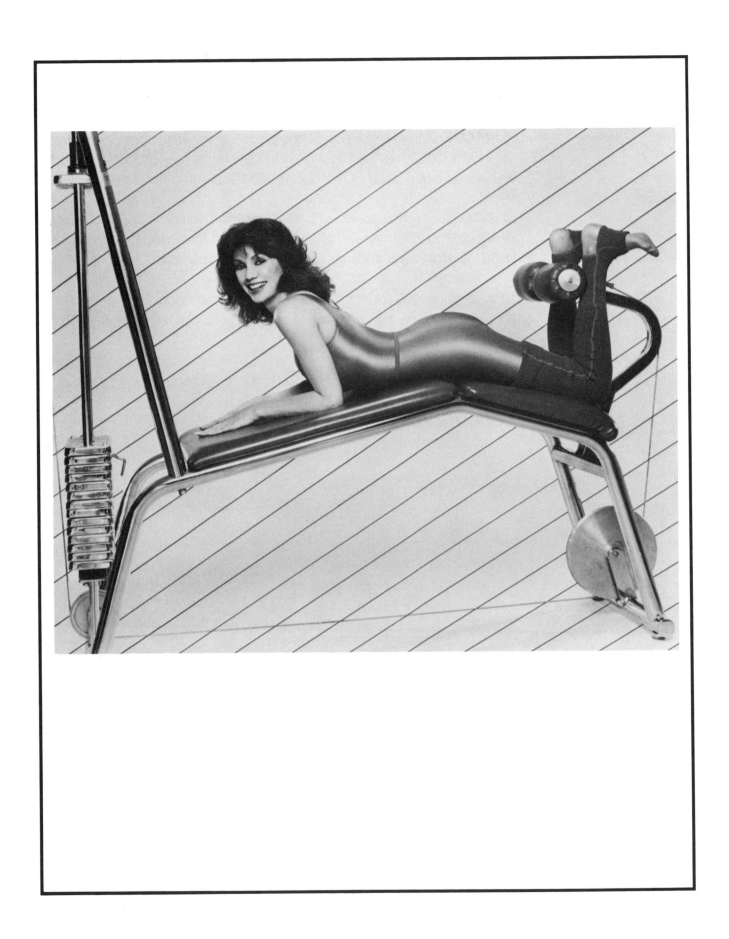

Pull-down

(BY UNIVERSAL)

PURPOSE: This exercise conditions the muscles of the upper and middle back and the fronts of the arms (the elbow flexors). Variations in the width and positioning of the hands will condition different fibers within those muscles.

MUSCLES: Middle and lower back (latissimus dorsi), upper back (shoulder girdle muscles) and fronts of the arms and forearms (elbow flexors)

TIME: Do for 30 seconds, as many as you can up to 15.

1. In a sitting position, grasp the bar above your head.
2. Pull down the bar in front of you to your shoulders, then let it back up.
3. Then pull it down again in back of your head to shoulder level. Repeat, continuously, in a smooth motion, without jerking the bar.

Repetitions: 15

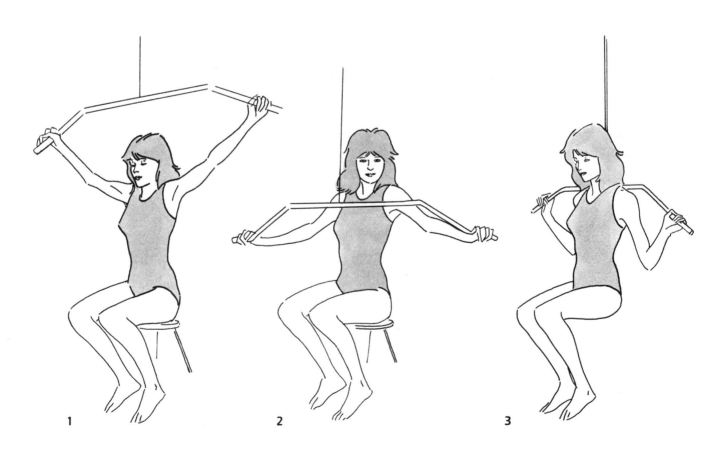

1   2   3

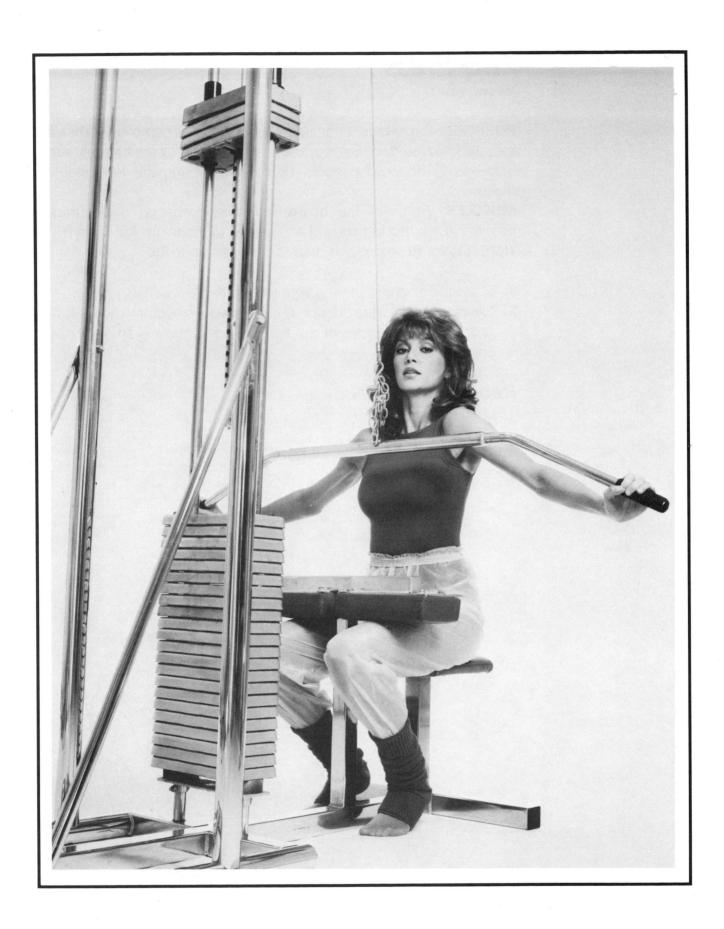

Leg Press

(BY UNIVERSAL)

PURPOSE: This exercise conditions the total hip/leg complex. Make sure the seat is adjusted so that your knees are well bent at the bottom of the movement. The weight should be moved through the full range of motion.

MUSCLES: Fronts of the thighs (quadriceps), backs of the thighs (hamstrings), buttocks (gluteals) and insides of the thighs (adductors)

TIME: Do for 30 seconds, as many as you can up to 15.

1. Sit on the machine, placing your feet on the foot pedals.
2. Extend your legs straight out in front of you, smoothly and carefully. Then bring your knees in toward you, again moving smoothly and continuously.

Repetitions: 15

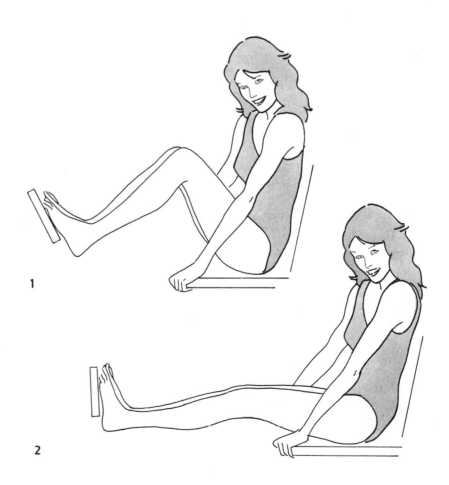

1

2

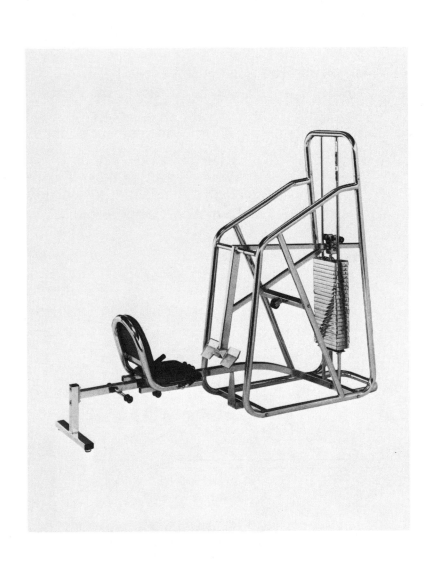

Chest Press

(BY UNIVERSAL)

PURPOSE: This exercise conditions the chest, the fronts of the shoulders and the backs of the arms. The grip may vary from narrow to wide, the most usual being a little wider than the shoulders.

MUSCLES: Fronts of the shoulders (anterior deltoids), chest (pectoralis major) and backs of the arms (triceps)

TIME: Do for 30 seconds, as many as you can up to 15.

1. Lie back on the bench with your feet on the floor, your hands gripping the bar above you.
2. Push up your arms as straight as possible (your elbows are straight, arms fully extended) and return to the starting position. Don't stop and don't jerk the motion. Complete it fully.

Repetitions: 15

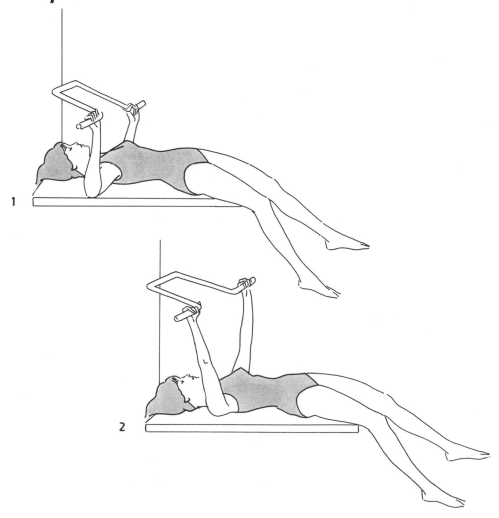

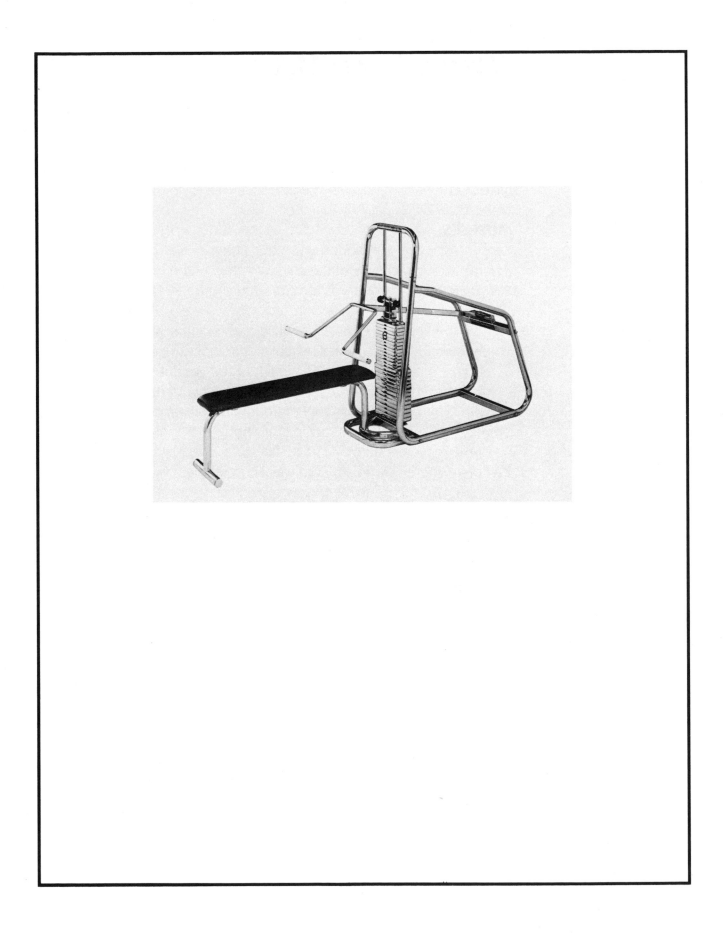

Rotary Torso Machine

(BY NAUTILUS)

PURPOSE: This exercise machine conditions the muscles that rotate your torso, sometimes called the "trunk." This is done by twisting the upper body against a fixed lower body and then repositioning the body for movement in the opposite direction. It makes certain that both sides of the body are equally conditioned.

MUSCLES: Muscles on the sides of the abdomen (external obliques), deep muscles on the abdominal sides (internal obliques) and muscles that run along each side of the spine (rotators of the trunk)

TIME: Do for 30 seconds, as many as you can up to 15.

1. Face the front of the machine while standing (the weight stack should be in back). Place the seat yoke (the adjustment is underneath) approximately 90 degrees to the left of the weight stack. Straddle the seat and cross your ankles securely. Don't let your hips and legs move with your body. Turn to the left, put your forearms on the pads and grasp the vertical bars. Your palms should be firmly against the bars of the movement arm.

2. Rotate your body (torso) from the left to the right by pushing your left palm. Use the trunk rotators to move the machine; your arms act as energy translators. Your head should move with your torso in one movement, with your eyes focusing between the vertical bars of the movement arm. (Sound complicated? Once you start it, it really is quite simple!) Rotate as far as possible for you, as long as you are not straining, and then return slowly to the starting position. Now repeat. For the reverse (right-to-left rotation), adjust the yoke to the opposite side of the machine and reverse the procedure.

Repetitions: 15

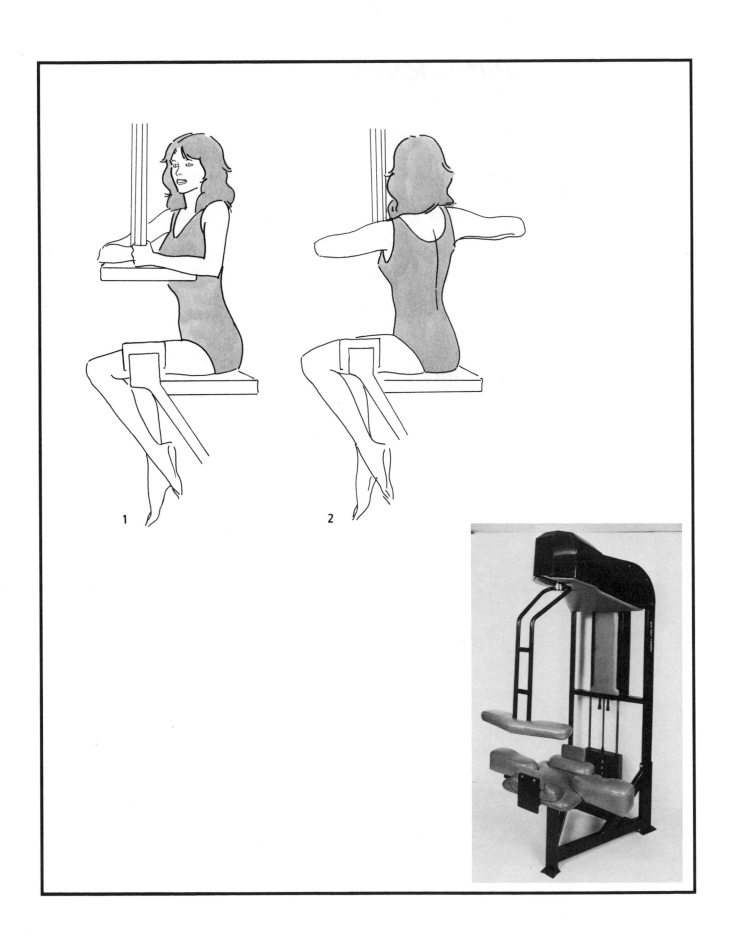

1

2

Push-down

(BY UNIVERSAL)

PURPOSE: This exercise conditions the extensor muscles of the elbow joint.

MUSCLES: Backs of the arms (triceps) and backs of the upper forearms (anconei)

TIME: Do for 30 seconds, as many as you can until 15.

1. Stand facing the machine and grasp the bar with an overhand grip.
2. Push down the bar until your arms are straight—completely extended. Hold your elbows close to your sides. Then bring your forearms back up. Repeat—smoothly and carefully, never jerking or stopping in the middle of the movement.

Repetitions: 15

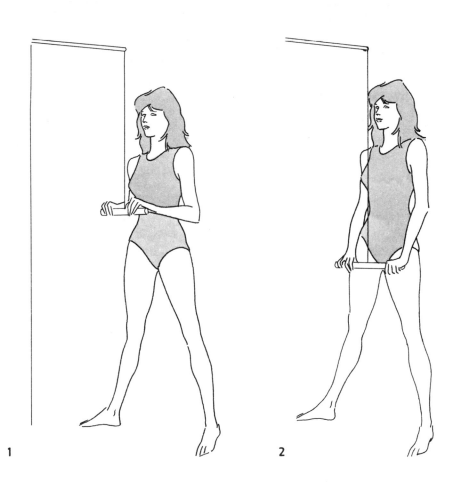

1   2

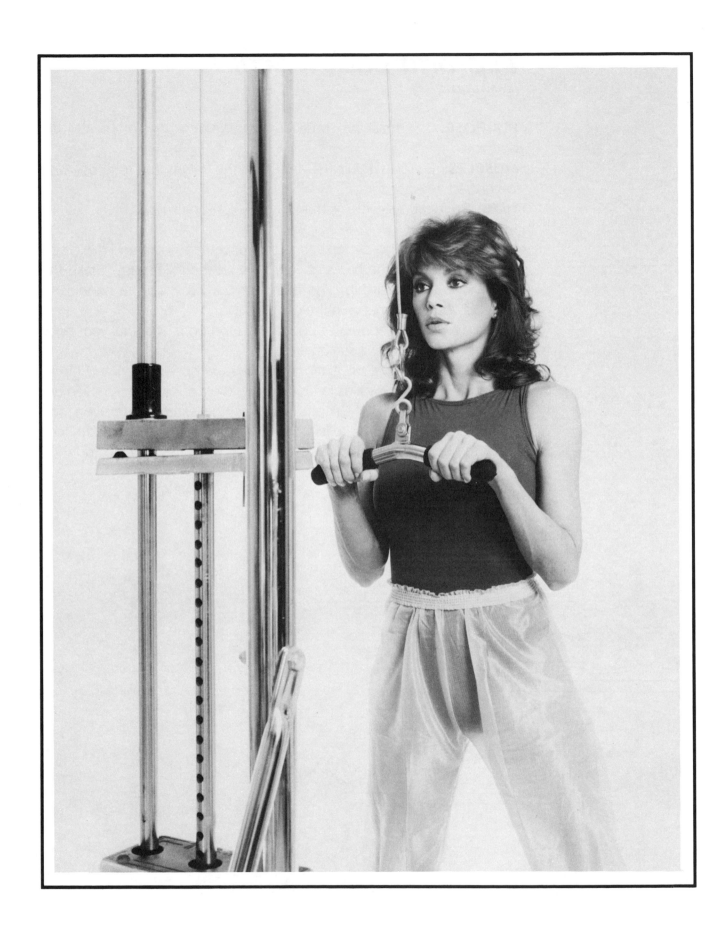

Hip-and-Back Machine

(BY NAUTILUS)

PURPOSE: This machine conditions the backs of the thighs and the buttocks.

MUSCLES: Buttocks (gluteals), backs of the thighs (hamstrings), and lower back (erector spinae)

TIME: Do for 30 seconds, as many as you can up to 15.

1. Enter the machine by separating the movement arms, and recline on your back with the backs of your legs on the roller pads. Grasp the handles near your hips and pull your body toward the handles to align your hip joints with the cams.

2. From a bent-hip and -knee position, extend both legs until your body and your legs form a straight line.

3. Holding one leg at full extension, allow the opposite leg and hip to bend and come back as far as possible. Work through the movement without stopping or jerking. Return to the extended position and repeat with the opposite leg. To get off the machine, bring both legs to the bent position (knees to the chest); separate the legs, and then slide out.

Repetitions: 15

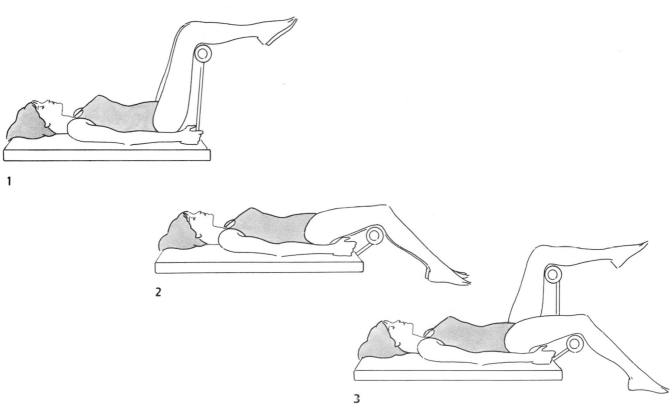

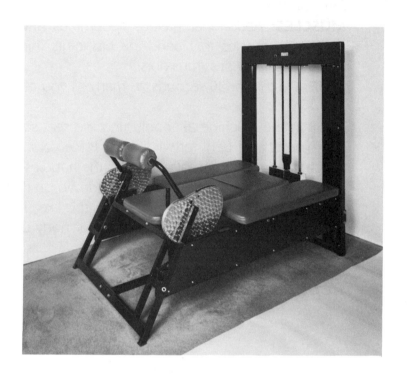

Abdominal Machine

(BY NAUTILUS)

PURPOSE: This exercise primarily conditions the abdominals, but it also strengthens the muscles that bend the hip joints and those under the arms on the sides of the chest.

MUSCLES: Abdominals (rectus abdominus and external and internal obliques), muscles that bend the hip joints (hip flexors), and muscles under the arms (latissimus dorsi)

TIME: Do this for 30 seconds, as many as you can up to 15.

1. Sit in the machine after adjusting the seat so that the middle of the spine can be bent forward easily. Place your ankles under the round pads beneath the seat and grasp the handles with both hands.

2. Begin your movement by pulling down on the handles while at the same time lifting with your legs. (Is this like chewing gum and walking at the same time?) Unbend your body until your back is in the original position. Then repeat again.

Repetitions: 15

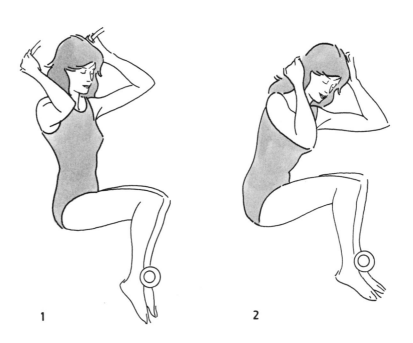

1   2

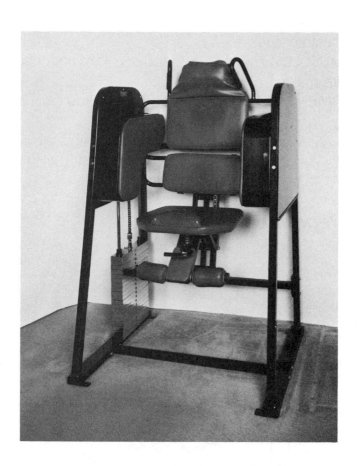

Vertical Fly

(BY UNIVERSAL)

PURPOSE: This exercise conditions the front of the shoulder area and the chest.

MUSCLES: Fronts of the shoulders (anterior deltoids) and chest (pectoralis major)

TIME: Do for 30 seconds, as many as you can up to 15.

1. Sit with your arms and forearms against the vertical pads.
2. Then swing your arms forward until the two pads come together. Repeat the movement. Smooth and easy—don't jerk.

Repetitions: 15

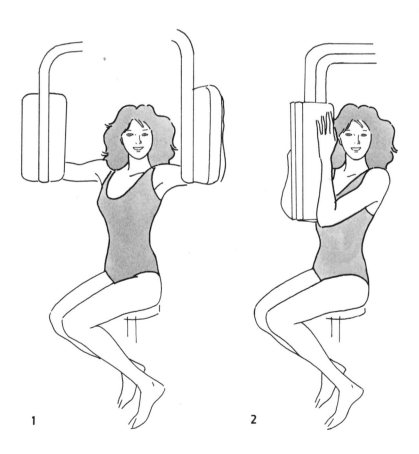

1   2

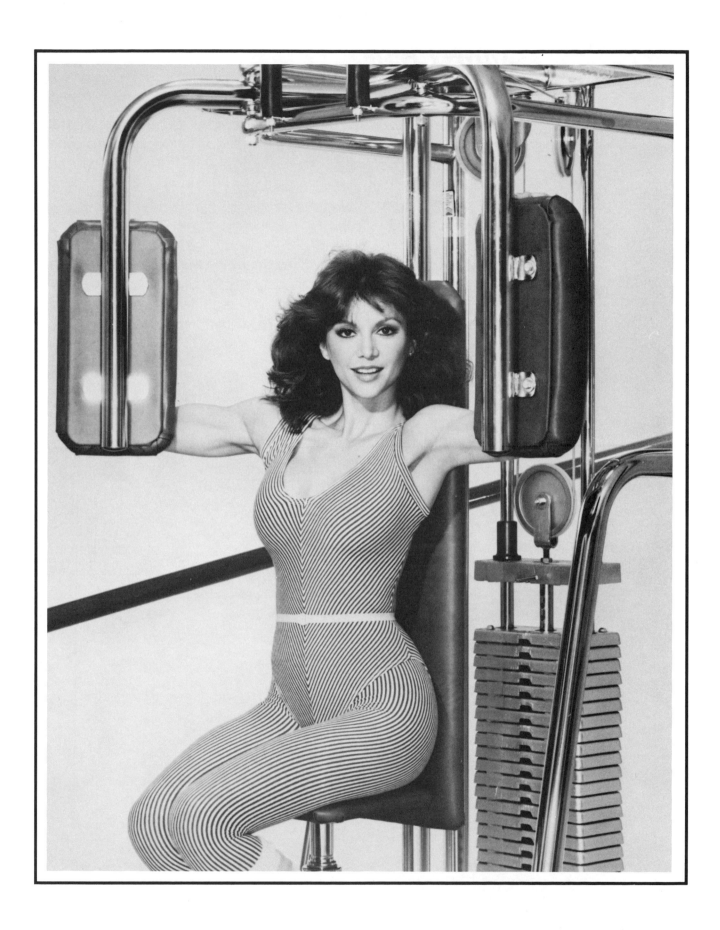

High Chair
(BY PARAMOUNT)

PURPOSE: This exercise conditions the muscles that bend the hips by lifting the legs and the lower abdominals. If done properly, it also conditions the lower abdominals.

MUSCLES: Those that lift the legs (hip flexors) and the long thin muscle of the stomach (restus abdominus)

TIME: Do this for 30 seconds, as many times as you can up to 15.

1. Rest your forearms on the armrests and grip the handles.
2. Bend your knees and then raise your hips by lifting your lower trunk and bringing your knees toward your shoulders. If you try to touch your knees to your shoulders, your lower abdominals will get a good workout.

Repetitions: 15

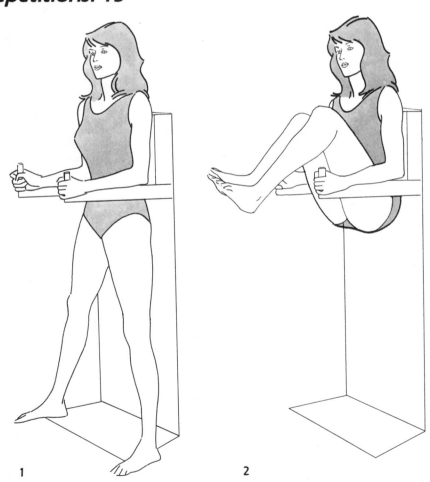

1   2

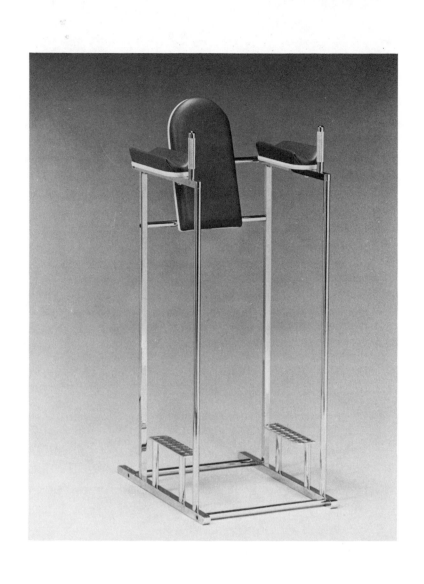

CHAPTER 6

The 30-Day Diet for Life

SENSIBLE IS BEST

I consider my body my most valuable possession—a machine, if you will—and thus the food I put into it has to be the best of all possible fuels and nutrients. I choose to give my body nourishing food (with only an occasional sinful dish) rather than pollute it with what I consider to be "poisons." After all, what's the point of exercising, toning my body, making it look and feel the best it can, if I then ruin it with unhealthy food?

It has been clear to me for a long time that all the exercise in the world will be for naught if I abuse my body by eating unhealthy food. We really are what we eat, in more ways than one. The food I digest affects my health, my energy, my temperament, my outlook on life. It also affects my body—how it looks, how it works, how it feels and how long it is going to be around.

Mark Twain once said, "Part of the secret of success in life is to eat what you like and let the food fight it out inside." But we know better. Nowadays, more and more people watch what and how much they eat. The choice, after all, is ours.

We've all read about the importance of eating well-balanced, nourishing meals. We know that foods with additives are not good for us; that too much salt affects our blood pressure and increases water retention; that fats cause unwanted amounts of cholesterol in the body; and that eating too much results in excessive and often unwanted fat. Sometimes all this information about the dangers of some foods and advice on what to do is confusing and overwhelming. For every theory on food and the body there is an expert who will agree with it or refute it. There is good cholesterol and bad cholesterol. You need some minerals, but an excess of one can cause an insufficiency of others. Vitamins are necessary but

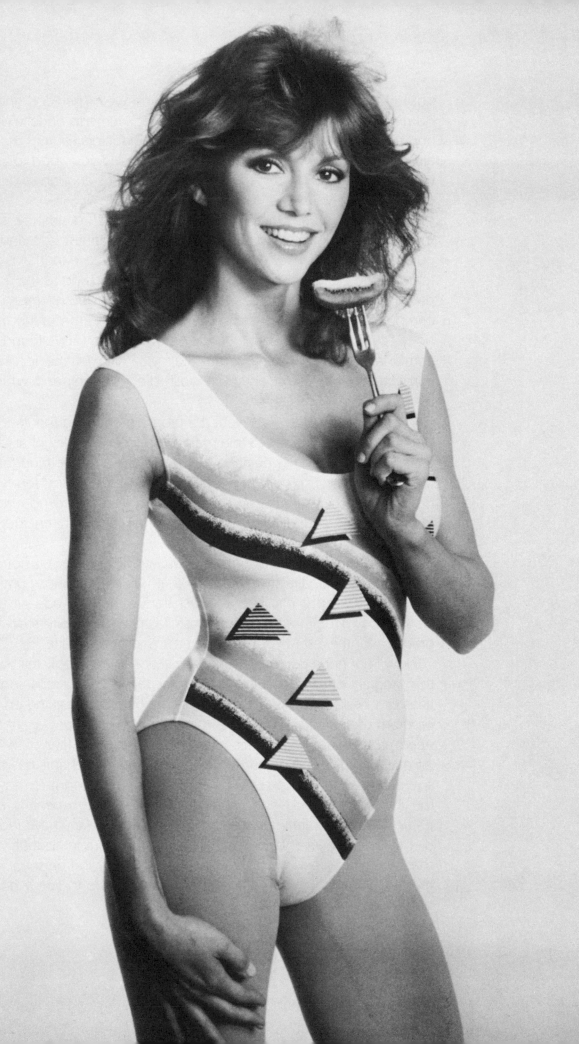

not if they are used as a substitute for eating well. The Food and Drug Administration suggests certain minimum requirements of daily vitamins and nutrients, but not everyone (not even the doctors!) agrees that these are correct. When was the last time you weighed your food to check if you were getting FDA minimum requirements? It's enough to drive you either to gorge yourself or to fast.

I do neither. I have tried, throughout the years, to simplify it all for myself. I have discussed diets and nutrition with physicians and many nutritionists. I have read a great deal about the subject and have gained (pardon the expression) a knowledge of what foods do to my body. By paying attention to every bit of food I eat (that doesn't mean being compulsive about it—just noting what it is that I am putting into my body), by watching to see the effects of these foods, I have found which combinations of foods make me healthy, which let me lose weight comfortably and permanently (no crash diets for me!) and which just plain do me wrong.

In the process, I have developed a program of eating that has let me lose weight when I want to and maintain my desired weight at all other times. It is a program of nutrition that has worked for me (and for many of my friends and coworkers who have tried it) for the last four years. It is a diet that is easy to follow, simple to eat (even at a friend's house or in a restaurant) and effective. It has made my body lean, energetic, and healthy.

I call the diet for losing weight the 30-Day Diet for Life. It is not a crash diet but a sensible life style of eating that will help you lose unwanted weight and keep it off. After the first thirty days, you add all but the "forbidden foods" (more about those later) and happily stay on this program for the rest of your life—a better and healthier life.

Now I am not a doctor, nor am I a nutritionist. I can only tell you how this program of eating healthy foods in certain combinations and quantities has helped me. And I do believe that before embarking on a *new* program of nutrition—whether it is to eat better or to lose weight—you need professional advice. Just as you would go to a lawyer for advice on a legal problem, a dentist for your teeth and a mechanic for your car, so I would urge you to see a doctor and/or a nutritionist for advice on the foods you should and should not eat to have a healthy body— particularly if you are interested in losing weight. Many have found my diet to be the perfect balanced eating program. But individuals are just that—individuals—with different health problems and personal characteristics. So make it really safe for yourself. Be sure to see a doctor or nutritionist first.

MODERATION AND BALANCE: THE SECRET TO NUTRITION

They say Mae West believed that "too much of a good thing is ecstasy." Food may be the only exception. Now I do not believe in living a life of total denial. I don't feel guilty if I take a bite out of a hamburger; I don't reproach myself if I eat a slice of chocolate pie; I haven't vowed that a slice of pizza will never pass my lips. Yet I do believe that eating any of these things excessively or regularly can be detrimental. My theory is that if I leave out the *very* bad foods, occasionally eat the questionable foods, and try to concentrate on eating the healthy foods, I'll be ahead of the game by far. The secret—the key—is moderation and balance.

But before you can balance the foods in your diet, you have to understand what your body needs to function successfully, and why it is that certain foods are just plain bad for you and should be eliminated from your diet. According to Sandy J. Wickham, who wrote a good book called *Human Nutrition: A Self-Instructional Text,* nutrition studies have shown "that greater familiarity with different foods and use of sound principles promote behavioral change and . . . development of beneficial food habits." In other words, if we understand how our bodies function, we will be more careful of the things we put into them.

I do believe that she is right. Every time I look at a slice of salami or bologna, I see those little pieces of fat clogging up my arteries and making themselves right at home on my thighs. I can't remember the last time I even considered eating a slice of salami.

FOOD IS FUEL

For the body, food is fuel, which enables it to function. Dr. Paul Ward explains it this way: "The body uses food in two ways: one, as a source of fuel for body heat, metabolism, muscular activity and work; and two, as a source of nutrients for continual repair and maintenance of all tissues. All foods can be used as fuel for energy, but no one food provides all the nutrients needed by the body." This is where balancing your foods comes in.

The body needs the "big six"—the basic nutrients found in food. They are: vitamins, minerals, proteins, fats, carbohydrates and water. Simply put, when digested and metabolized, these nutrients interact with the enzymes and coenzymes in our bodies to produce, among other things, energy. The *vitamins* in our system regulate this metabolic process and help build up tissues and bones. They are found in foods and can also be taken in the form of a food supplement (the vitamin pill). *Minerals*, also found in the foods we eat (particularly in vegetables and meats), act to regulate chemical reactions in our cells and are important for adequate muscle contraction in the body. Potassium, calcium, magnesium, iodine and iron are some of the minerals our bodies must have.

Proteins are everywhere in our bodies. According to Dr. Ward: "Protein contains many amino acids which are the basic building blocks for tissue maintenance, growth and repair. It makes up the cell membranes and nuclei. . . . The blood contains proteins, and the amino acids in the protein serve as the basic building blocks for hormones and enzymes." Although it is the proteins from animals (meats) which are said to provide those essential amino acids in the right proportion for use in the body, proteins from vegetables can be combined in a way to effectively nourish us.

Then there are *fats* (and you thought you only wanted to get rid of fat!). Contrary to what we may have thought, fats are essential for the functioning of our bodies. Besides insulating us from the cold, fats serve as a source of energy and carry certain vitamins throughout our system. *Carbohydrates* are also essential to our bodies since they are our main source of fuel. We get carbohydrates from cereals, fruits, vegetables, pasta and breads. Our central nervous system operates almost exclusively on carbohydrates; thus a lack of an adequate supply would limit endurance in exercise and also hamper the functioning of our nervous system. Lest you get carried away with the sudden importance of noodles in your life, you should know that there are two kinds of carbohydrates. Explains Dr. Ward: "Nutritionists often divide carbohydrates into two groups—natural, or 'complex,' carbohydrates (the 'good' guys) and processed, or 'refined,' carbohydrates (the 'bad' guys). The complex carbohydrates (found in fruits and vegetables and whole-grain products) are more desirable because they convert into blood sugar slowly and supply us with vitamins, minerals and roughage. The bad guys—those in colas and white breads and sugary cereals—are essentially empty calories and low in nutritional value. Because they are converted into glucose rapidly, they cause blood sugar imbalances and are responsible for lots of different ailments (from tooth decay to diabetes to heart disease)."

Finally there is *water*—without which the body cannot survive. Water is needed for nearly all our body processes (60 percent of your body weight is water) and is especially important for temperature regulation. Water, explains Sandy Wickham, "is the medium in which body chemical reactions occur and is the transporter of necessary materials to the cells and metabolic wastes from the cells." Water is found in our taps and in bottles (*note*: I drink Saratoga Naturally Sparkling Mineral Water—it is salt free) and also in fruits and vegetables. But the body needs more water than you can find in these foods, so, yes, you do need to drink at least eight glasses of it a day (it's easier than you think—see page 176).

RULES TO EAT BY

Back to balancing. The basic idea behind having a diet made up of well-balanced meals, whether it is to lose weight or to maintain it—is to make sure you eat enough basic "good" foods which have sufficient nutrients to make you healthy. This is more serious (and probably less complicated) than you may think. You probably know that women's bodies need iron, particularly since we lose it monthly during menstruation, and that to get it we need to eat beans, eggs, green leafy vegetables, whole grains and organic meats (no hormones). You probably also have heard that calcium affects bones and teeth, muscles and nerve tissues, and that by eating broccoli, some dairy products, salmon, watercress and almonds, you will ensure that your body gets its requirement of calcium. But do you spend time worrying about your intake of potassium (did you even know that a deficiency in potassium can cause muscle weakness, cramps, irritability?). Do you keep a count of how many calories you eat every day? Do you measure and weigh the foods you eat to know how much of what nutrient you are giving your body?

I don't. It is impossible to carry on a productive and full life, to enjoy yourself, and at the same time measure and weigh everything you eat. Very few people have the extraordinary discipline necessary to keep up with compulsive measuring and note keeping about what you should and should not have. And it is unnecessary. The point is not to memorize charts of which vitamins and minerals are in which foods. Rather, we can easily balance our meals by leaving out harmful foods and trying to eat a little of each of the good ones.

The easiest way to reeducate oneself about eating a good balanced diet is to know which foods are the harmful ones. By merely cutting these foods out of my diet, I know I am not polluting my body.

FORBIDDEN FOODS

There are some foods I never eat. Not only when I am on a weight-reduction program—*never*. Now remember: Falling off the good-nutrition wagon is not fatal; so by never I don't mean that eating a slice of pizza once every other month is grounds for self-flagellation! Rather, I have made it a point to *try* to stay away from certain foods.

Some things just aren't worth it. Like salt. Do yourself a favor—give it up. Salt causes water retention and is disastrous for your blood pressure, among other things. There is nothing good about adding salt (sodium chloride) to your foods—it's already in almost everything we eat in much larger quantities than we need. Medical experts seem to agree that we don't need more than 3,000 milligrams (that's 3 grams) of sodium per day. If that sounds like a lot, wait until you hear how much is already in the foods many of us eat regularly! One Big Mac has 1,500 milligrams of sodium. One teaspoon of salt has more than 2,000 milligrams. Three ounces of mayonnaise has 600 milligrams. Salt is in cottage cheese, soy sauce, in tuna packed in oil, in canned chicken broth and tomato sauce, in breads—in almost everything.

Thus the point is that if you try to cut out most of these foods, and substitute other similar products for the salted ones (eat unsalted almonds and wheat pretzels; drink salt-free Saratoga mineral water; season with Worcestershire sauce instead of soy; make your own broth with a salt substitute rather than buying canned broth), you'll be way ahead of the game. Try preparing your meals without salt—you'll find that you are, for the first time, really *tasting* the food you have cooked, and, after a couple of weeks, I guarantee you'll find you don't miss the salt at all.

There is no real salt at my house. My shakers are full of a salt substitute called Neocurtasal (I buy it at my local pharmacy). Being the only cook in my house (and I love to cook!), I have served countless dinner guests saltless meals where the tabletop saltshakers were full of Neocurtasal and there was no salt in the food—and no one has ever noticed.

Another no-no is cheese. Cheese is concentrated fat; if you insist on eating it, you might as well spread it on your thighs. That's surely where it will show up anyway, sooner than later. Although low-fat cheese is better, no cheese is best. It sounds radical—but believe me, eating some of these foods is merely a habit. Once you break it, you forget. Once I stopped eating cheese, I forgot about it. (I remember eating a slice of pizza some months later and thinking, "What's the big deal? It's not that great!") The only cheese I eat is grated Parmesan cheese packaged in a container—the kind you find at any supermarket. I use it as a spice to season various dishes.

Other milk products are also not on my diet. I drink only low-fat milk (on the thirty-day reducing program I drink no milk or only nonfat milk). Plain low-fat yogurt (the flavored ones are full of sugar) is better than regular yogurt. I put "regular" yogurt on my skin for facials because the skin absorbs the fat in the yogurt—fat my body doesn't need. Low-fat yogurt is a terrific substitute for sour cream; try it on baked potatoes or on a chicken taco. It is delicious!

Then there is butter. I have gotten so used to eating without butter that I don't even use margarine. Butter is pure fat, and my body has no use for it. Neither does it want mayonnaise; it is full of salt *and* fat. A little now and then is okay, but get into the habit of using low-fat yogurt instead. Believe me, I don't miss any of these fats! I look and feel great without them in and on my body—and food tastes just as good without them, if not better.

I stay away from anything with the word cream in it. Cream cheese, whipped cream, ice cream (okay—every now and then), cream dressings, cream soups, sour cream—just substitute the word fat for cream (ice fat, fat cheese, whipped fat) and giving it up will be quite easy.

I also stay away from any foods that end in "ami"—salami, pastrami, bologna (well, sort of). And "eef"—roast beef, corned beef, smoked beef, pepper beef. You get the point. Obviously I am not alone in condemning red meat. It's the one thing almost all medical experts agree on: Red meat is just not good for you. I stopped eating it about five years ago, and I don't miss it a bit. I really feel somehow cleaner without it. (My eating program will clean out your body. It will rid it of toxins. You'll notice your skin become beautifully translucent, and your energy level will rise significantly.) But if you find that you need a little red meat once in a while, try eating it not more than once a week. And make it veal, which has the least fat of the red meats.

Again, I'm not advocating total denial. Most people get depressed when asked to stop eating things they love, and then they get discouraged from trying the diet. I myself was intimidated by giving up red meat entirely. So I left myself one form of it—bacon. I treat myself to bacon for breakfast once every other week. Since that's my only intake of meat, it hasn't seemed to harm me at all.

We should tackle fried foods. I'm sure you've already heard all you want to hear about the drawbacks of frying foods. Again, fat is the villain. It's been years since I've eaten fried foods (except for that bacon), yet I still remember feeling so greasy after I ate anything fried—it was an awful feeling. Now I broil or steam or bake those same foods. I used to eat French fries; now I eat baked, steamed or boiled potatoes with pepper and low-fat yogurt, parsley or dill, and a dab of margarine occasionally—delicious! I used to eat fried fish. Now, it's baked fish wrapped in tinfoil, smothered in onions and green peppers, scallions, dill, white wine—a favorite at my house. Serve it with rice (pour the sauce from the fish over it) and steamed vegetables. Get the idea?

If the loss of these forbidden foods is depressing you, give yourself a reward. After you complete the thirty-day diet and embark on your new lifetime healthy eating plan, indulge in a favorite dessert to take the edge off, or have that bacon once in a while. Whatever you miss, have it as a treat, in small amounts and rarely. But—trust me. After a while you'll be so used to eating healthy foods, and you'll feel so good, that you'll wonder how you could have ever abused your now wonderful body.

PRINCIPLES OF THE 30-DAY DIET FOR LIFE

Once you choose to embark on The 30-Day Diet for Life, you do so to lose weight and to start a whole new way of eating. You will almost assuredly lose anywhere from five to thirty pounds on this diet, easily and healthfully. Enjoy it! Don't weigh yourself every hour—once a week will do. After the thirty days are up, you continue your newly acquired eating habits, adding anything you want except for the forbidden foods (see the chart on page 183).

I eat a full breakfast every day on the maintenance plan. You'll often find me at the studio at 6:30 A.M. devouring one or two poached eggs, one slice of dry wheat toast (sometimes two), half a slice tomato and a cup of tea. Once a week I'll indulge in bacon or potatoes (not both). Again—only moderate denials. If, after another month or so, you want to lose additional weight, just return to the thirty-day plan. You can do so at any time. I have been on the lifetime diet for months, returned to the thirty-day diet and then gone back to the maintenance diet. Because this is not a crash program, but rather a sensible food plan resulting in a healthy and clean system, my body is never harmed, and my weight does not fluctuate drastically. As a matter of fact, for the last five years I have never fluctuated more than two pounds on either side of 110.

And, thus, the principles:

1. Get a twenty-five-cent spiral note pad/diary and write down every-thing you eat for the first seven days. Make a game out of it—write down every bit of food and how much you ate. At the end of the day, read it. You'll learn more about what your body is digesting than ever before, and after the week is over, you'll be able to see why (or why not) you lost weight.

2. Drink a glass of water before each meal (try to make it fifteen or thirty minutes before you eat) and a glass of iced tea with each meal. If you want a glass of sparkling water, make it salt free. You'll thus automatically have at least six glasses of water a day. Why iced tea? It is the perfect natural diuretic.

3. Eat the foods in the combinations I describe. Don't make your own substitutions until you are past the thirty-day plan. I have found that these combinations work together in your system to result in proper weight loss. So have that tomato *with* the toast, and follow the tuna with the iced tea.

4. Never ever eat after eight at night. The food you eat later will just sit in your stomach. Make breakfast your biggest meal, lunch moderate, and dinner your smallest.

5. Eat as much chicken as the program calls for. I have not specified quantities in weights because I don't believe most people weigh food (I never have!). When I say two slices, you know best how much you can and will eat. Just remember—no skin. And try to buy chicken that has not been treated with hormones. The reason some farmers inject their chickens with hormones is to make them fatter. You need neither the chemicals nor that extra fat in your body.

6. Eggs are allowed and encouraged on this food plan but never cooked in butter. If you have high cholesterol, ask your doctor about the egg allotment. (You can hard boil an egg and just eat the white on toast with tomatoes, if you like.) Eggs can be scrambled, poached, boiled and hard boiled all with water—no fat.

7. Eat wheat toast, preferably with fiber in it. Never eat toast after lunch time. And *do* eat it—don't think you are doing yourself a favor if you leave it out. Everything on this diet should be eaten as prescribed.

8. I don't think coffee is good for you. Besides its many detriments, caffeine buildup is especially dangerous for women who have a tendency to develop cysts. If you *must* have it, drink decaffeinated coffee and make it only a once-a-week deal. Get into the tea habit—either herbal or regular (you have to drink very strong tea in order to be affected by the caffeine in it).

9. Only nonfat milk during the first thirty days. If you have to have a touch in your tea, okay. But try not to. After the thirty days you can have low-fat or nonfat—but never again shall whole milk pass those lips. If you are worried about the calcium you may lose, eat broccoli (2½ cups equal a glass of milk) and take a calcium tablet three times a day. Talk to your doctor about vitamin supplements. I have taken them for years and am a great believer in them.

10. Veal, a red meat, has little fat in it. If you just love it, have it once a week during the thirty days. You can eat liver after the first thirty days but only once a month.

11. The following vegetables can be eaten during the thirty days (best steamed and dotted with seasonings, including grated Parmesan cheese— but never butter):

asparagus
broccoli (the perfect vegetable—has a lot of calcium and potassium)
brussels sprouts
cabbage (if you get gaseous, braise it or leave it out)
cauliflower (same as above)
celery (cooked—it has less salt in it this way)
chives
cucumber (hothouse—produces less gas)
eggplant
endive
garlic (also garlic powder for seasoning—never garlic salt)
green beans (they make a great snack when they are cold)
green pepper (cook with eggs for a healthy omelette)
lettuce
mushrooms
onions
parsley
potatoes (twice during the first month—steamed)
radishes
red cabbage
scallions
spinach (with lemon if it's not too acidic for you—no butter or margarine)
squash
tomatoes (actually a fruit)
watercress
zucchini

12. No canned food except for salmon and tuna packed in water. I am serious—no canned soups, no canned tomato sauce, no canned vegetables or fruits; they have too much sugar and salt. Go fresh!

13. No sugar cereals. The only cereal I eat is Cheerios—I have found it to be nutritious. Or, if you prefer, any seven-grain or oat cereal—hot or cold—is fine.

14. Very little fruit during the first thirty days (too much sugar). Melons and strawberries are okay. Oranges and grapefruit are all right but only if they are not too acidic for your system (only you can know). (If you find you have this problem take an antacid. It helps—and many brands have calcium in them.) If you find you have a regularity problem, eat fibrous bread and drink one glass of prune juice before breakfast. Again, check with your doctor or nutritionist about the advisability of taking vitamin supplements.

15. Use only low-cal salad dressings. Say goodbye to cream dressings of any kind. Aim for diet and/or low-sodium dressings. Try combining Japanese rice vinegar with a touch of Dijon mustard (no oil!).

16. Pasta is okay, but cook it without oil or salt. Rinse it after it is cooked in running water to get rid of the extra starch. Make a sauce with fresh tomatoes, Italian spices, green peppers, mushrooms, onions and lots of garlic—but no oil. Another great sauce is made with fresh vegetables.

17. No alcohol during the thirty days. Not even a lite beer (which is fine after the first month).

18. No pickled foods—pickles, relish. No ketchup. No syrups or sweets—not even raisins. No nuts at first. After thirty days, you can eat almonds and walnuts.

19. If you find yourself in a restaurant during the first thirty days, don't panic. There's a simple balancing act you can perform. Look at the menu and find the least objectionable items. Ask the chef to make a pasta sauce without oil, a salad with dressing on the side, or broiled fish. Iced tea is always available (remember—no sugar). After the thirty days, look at the menu with new eyes. If you can't pass up the pasta with garlic, have it. But then no dessert. If the zabaglione or white chocolate cake makes your heart beat faster (and it literally will), order it, but have a simple salad or broiled fish as a main course. Remember, balance, balance, balance, and you'll never feel cheated.

20. No diet sodas. After the thirty days, only if you have to, and only three a week. Drink your iced tea!

21. Eat three meals a day. Eat until you feel full. If you do need a snack, try munching on an apple—but after the thirty days. For those of you used to snacking, this will be the hardest part of this diet. But stick to the three-meals-a-day rule—it is worth it.

22. Learn to use seasonings freely. I put garlic on everything! (If you find you have garlic breath, an antacid will neutralize the acid in your stomach and reduce the odor.) Seasonings that I use include:

grated Parmesan cheese packaged in a container (the only cheese you are allowed forever)
celery powder
red pepper or black pepper
Italian herb mixture (in spaghetti sauce, naturally, but try it on a tomato-on-toast sandwich)
garlic powder
cinnamon
lemon bits
basil
sage
marjoram
dill
dry mustard
paprika
cloves
curry
ginger
nutmeg
sesame seeds
poppy seeds

SEVEN-DAY MENU*

MONDAY

Breakfast

1 egg (cooked any style but without butter)

1 slice of wheat toast, dry

½ tomato, sliced

tea (hot or cold, no sugar, no cream; you can have nonfat milk; lemon in the morning is too acidic)

or decaffeinated coffee (if you must)

Lunch

salad (no tomato)—include onions, any vegetables on the list, sliced turkey (not smoked); low-cal dressing

iced tea (no sugar—use artificial sweetener if you like)

Dinner

steamed vegetable platter—no butter or margarine; use grated Parmesan cheese flakes for seasoning, plus any spices you like. Combine any vegetables on the list.

iced tea

TUESDAY

Breakfast

1 juice glass of prune juice

½ melon (Crenshaw or cantaloupe)

1 slice wheat toast, dry

tea

Lunch

lettuce, tomato, tuna with low-cal dressing

iced tea

Dinner

1 cup chicken broth (make it yourself—no salt)

cooked celery

1 slice white-meat chicken

½ cup (cooked) brown rice

iced tea

*Repeat three times, then add the first two days for a total of thirty days. Start on a Monday; calling each day by a number gets confusing. Remember—one glass of water before each meal (try fifteen to thirty minutes before). Quantities, if not specified, are up to you (but don't eat a whole turkey at one sitting).

WEDNESDAY

Breakfast
whole tomato sliced on dry toast (with parsley or Italian seasoning)
tea

Lunch
chicken salad (no mayonnaise, no tomato; low-cal dressing)
2 Melba toasts
iced tea

Dinner
steamed vegetable platter (no Parmesan this time—use other seasonings; pick from any vegetables on the list)
iced tea

THURSDAY

Breakfast
1 juice glass of prune juice
1 egg
1 slice wheat toast, dry
½ tomato, sliced
tea

Lunch
vegetable platter (raw or steamed)
iced tea

Dinner
2 slices of veal, baked (may substitute chicken; no oil or butter)
1 vegetable, steamed (approx. 1 cup)
iced tea

FRIDAY

Breakfast
½ melon (slice of lemon okay)
1 slice wheat toast, dry
tea

Lunch
shrimp with sliced mushrooms, tomatoes on lettuce (low-cal dressing; if shrimp is not available, substitute tuna)
iced tea

Dinner
steamed vegetable platter (Use any seasonings you like)
iced tea

SATURDAY

Breakfast
1 cup strawberries (with nonfat milk, if you like)
and/or 1 cup Cheerios (you can combine the two and add artificial sweetener if you like; if you prefer, use a bran cereal)
tea

Lunch
salad—anything you like, plus tomato
1 Melba toast
iced tea

Dinner
chicken or turkey or veal
½ sliced tomato salad with low-cal dressing
iced tea
1 glass of wine if you like

SUNDAY

Breakfast
1 juice glass of prune juice
1 egg
1 slice wheat toast, dry
½ tomato sliced and/or 1 slice melon
tea
(If you like a Sunday brunch, combine the breakfast and lunch menus.)

Lunch
salad
iced tea

Dinner

broiled (or canned) salmon

½ cup pasta with boiled tomato sauce—make your own; no canned
allowed (can substitute two vegetables or 1 vegetable and 2 Melba
toasts if you don't want the pasta)

FOOD CHART

The 30-Day Diet for Life Foods	Forever Foods (After 30 Days)	Forbidden Foods (Almost Never)
	All foods on the 30-Day Diet plus the following additions:	
Nonfat milk	Low-fat milk	Cheese
Eggs	Potatoes	Milk products (except low-fat yogurt and nonfat and low-fat milk)
Wheat toast/Melba toast	Fruits and berries	
Tomatoes	Low-fat yogurt (Plain)	
Iced or hot tea (no sugar)	Fish and shellfish	Red meat and cured meat
Salads	Alcohol and lite beer	Olives
Low-cal dressings (never creamed)	Oatmeal	Salt
	Unsalted nuts	Butter
Vegetables (see page 178)	Unsalted crackers	Avocados
Turkey and chicken	Wheat pretzels (no salt)	Mayonnaise
Veal (optional)	Bacon (occasionally and only if you love it)	Cola drinks (diet okay now and then)
Shrimp		
Grated Parmesan cheese	Breads (stick to fibers)	Soy sauce
Seasonings (see page 179)	Sauces (if you make them yourself and no cream ever!)	Potato chips and pretzels
Melon (not watermelon)		Oil
Chicken broth (homemade, no salt)	Jams (no preservatives, low sugar)	Peanut butter and peanuts
		Sugar cereals
Tuna and salmon (fresh or canned in water)	Vegetables-and-pasta soups (make them yourself)	White rice
Strawberries		Candy and other excessive sugars
Cheerios (or any seven-grain or oat cereal) or bran cereal		Honey
		Canned anything
Pasta		Pizza
Brown rice		
Prune juice		

IT WORKS

The 30-Day Diet for Life works. That's the most exciting thing about it. It works—quickly, easily, healthfully. The first thirty days are the key; if you stick to the diet, you'll lose the weight and you will probably never put it back on. And, if you get into the habit of eating this way, the "rest of your life" program, with its many delicious additions, will be a breeze. Challenge yourself—*choose* to make yourself healthy and fit. You've already chosen to make The Body Principal Program of exercise a routine part of your life. Add The Body Principal "Eating for Life" Plan, and you're on your way to making the best you possible. The 30-Day Diet for Life plan sets you up for an eating program that will last forever.

And there it is—a philosophy of moderation and balance, a careful selection of foods that helps you remain healthy, and, when combined with The Body Principal Program of exercise, will result in that permanently wonderful-looking and -feeling you.

CHAPTER 7

A Life Style of Maintenance

PHYSICAL AND MENTAL HARMONY

For me, exercising is not merely something I do to look more attractive. Making The Body Principal Program a way of life has meant not only that my body looks the way I want it to, but that I feel wonderful inside.

I have always felt that the body and the mind are one. Recent research has shown that physical fitness is an excellent way to alleviate stress as well as some types of depression. If your body is in shape, you will feel better. The way we think and feel has a direct effect on the body—every nerve, every muscle. Likewise, the shape we are in affects our mental well-being. I believe the two are inseparable and that to create internal peace, we need to create physical peace as well. The way to do that is to exercise.

Exercise releases the stress and tension of our daily lives, while at the same time releasing energy that results in progress. Motion is progress. If you develop and take care of your body, you cannot stagnate. It is hard to be lethargic while doing fifty calf exercises on the stairs to the theme from *Star Wars;* it is difficult (if not impossible) to be unhappy and tense while tightening your thighs to Donna Summer. Emotional tension and stress—which when stored in your body can affect your heart, circulatory system, blood pressure, and muscles—are released in exercise. As you do The Body Principal Program, as you work those muscles, your blood rushes through your body. You work hard and you feel energized, ready to move. It is difficult to remain lazy or depressed when you exercise—particularly when you see the results you have been striving for and you begin to enjoy the process of exercising.

Stress is a part of all our lives. It shows up in various guises—as sleeplessness, irritability, illness, lack of concentration, and in many other ways. It is a dangerous force that, if not released, causes depression and unhappiness at the least, coronaries and strokes and even death at the worst. It is present, in various degrees, in all of us. Even in the best of times, you can still retain stress in your body. Sometimes people say to me, "Victoria, everything is going your way. You are successful, you have a nice home and friends and a career—how can you feel stressful?" But no matter how happy you are, everyday tensions are a fact of life.

I have learned to deal with stress by using The Body Principal Program. Besides exercising every day, throughout the day, I also use the exercises as a tool to fight the tension and stress in my daily life. Here is a recent example, which happened while we were shooting the exercise photographs for this book.

Conflicting and full schedules—mine and Harry Langdon's, the photographer for this book (and my friend)—meant that we had to shoot them while I was also filming "Dallas." (This was at a time when the character I play, Pam, had a lot of crises in her life, which meant I had a lot of lines to learn.) I managed to take off a few days to shoot these photographs. The days were fun—but long. The sessions started at 7:30 in the morning and ended around 8 at night. By the third day, I arrived feeling tired, tense—absolutely burnt out.

It is an awful feeling. If you have ever woken up in the morning and felt you just could not function, that's what I call "stressed out." Anger and frustration and fatigue build up inside until finally your body cannot cope. Someone on the set said, "You look tired. Let me rub your neck." And I, who love neck rubs, answer, "No, thank you." I can't be touched—I am raw from head to toe. I feel as though all my nerve endings are on fire. That is stressed out. My mind and body shut down, saying, "Victoria, we've had enough."

That day at Harry's studio I was under that strain. Then I started warming up to exercise for the photographs. Soon I was going through The Body Principal Program—the calf exercises up and down on the stairs, the thigh pulls on the mat, the leg lifts and the running. The more I worked my body, the better I felt. Suddenly, I not only forgot about my depression, I began to feel energized, excited, almost high. My body was working—I was moving and feeling elated, and the stress and tension just disappeared. My body and my mind were in harmony. It reminded me, right then and there, of how much a part of my life exercise had become, and what a wonderful tool it is to aid in physical and emotional happiness. As long as my body is in shape, my mind works at its full capacity. I get more oxygen to my brain. I move easier, with energy flowing through me. Suddenly I am thinking more clearly, responding quickly. I am able to focus, to concentrate on whatever I am doing.

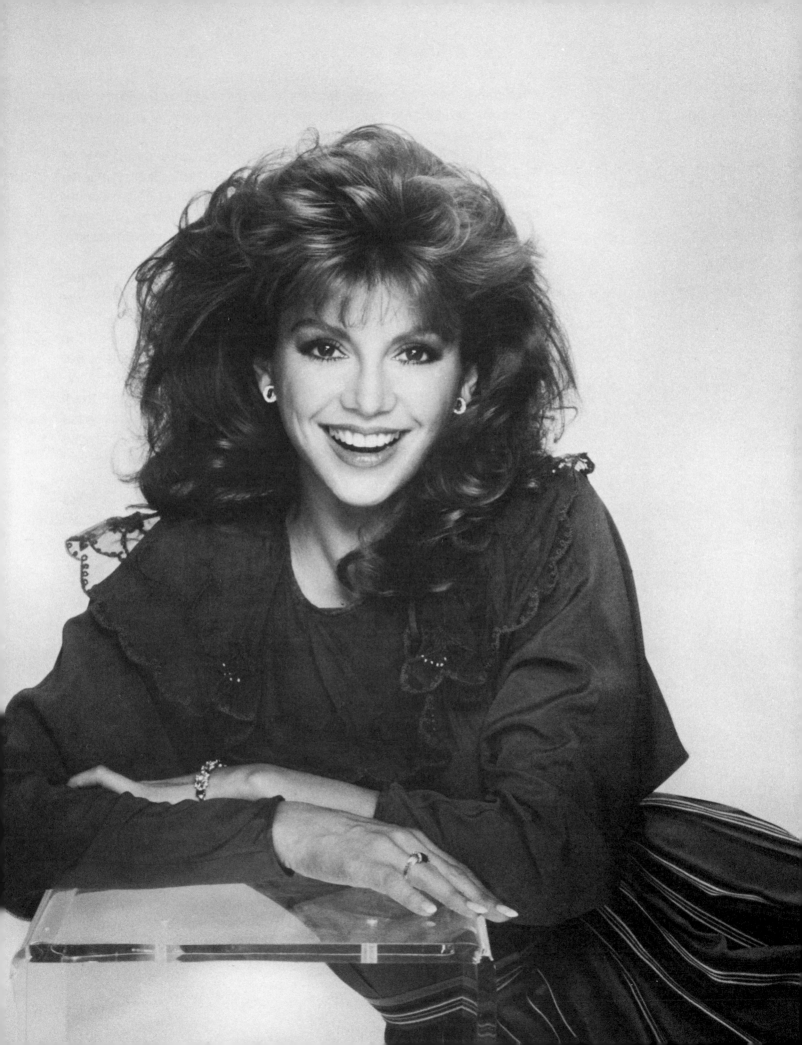

Everything seems somehow simpler, more clear-cut, manageable. My emotions flourish; the stress disappears. I am a happy and productive person once more.

This kind of stress happens to everyone. All our daily schedules, no matter what our life styles or professions, are to some extent, at some time, too hectic to handle with ease. When you get up early to make breakfast, take the kids to school, prepare for work, put in a full day at the office, then return home to care for others or go out to entertain a client or friends, that is hectic and often stressful.

I have learned that I can stop the cycle of built-up tension, fatigue, and unhappiness due to stress: I do my exercises throughout the day. Sometimes on the set I go into a corner or to the ladies' room and do my resistive exercises for a full five minutes. Then I either take a catnap right then and there or put my head down on a desk for another five minutes. You'll be surprised at the difference that can make!

If you have a ten-minute coffee break, take the break and give them back the coffee. Exercise for five minutes and then rest for five. Instead of giving in to the stress and the caffeine, turn to your body. It will always be there—and it will always come through for you.

And, at the end of the day, rather than putting on more makeup so you'll look better, do some exercises and take another nap or a quick bath. You'll feel better *and* look better. Then, when you go out to dinner and people say, "Don't tell me you went to work today—you look fabulous," you can simply smile.

Exercising does not mean that you will never again feel stress or tension. It does mean that you will be more resistant to stress and will be able to quickly alleviate it. I don't believe that doing resistive exercises will solve all your problems, but I can assure you that in my experience, these exercises, besides toning and resculpting your body, cleanse your head and energize you so you can better cope with that daily stress.

I have found, and this I firmly believe, that if you have a healthy and happy body, it will be a better home for that intangible but very precious thing—your soul.

SEX AND EXERCISE

The Body Principal Program affects many parts of your life. It not only results in a resculpted, toned, stronger body and in a less stressful, more harmonious union between body and mind, it also makes you a more productive, energetic person and can improve the quality of your sex life.

Let me explain. The first effect resistive exercising has on your sex life is that exercising the muscles used in sexual intercourse strengthens and tones them. This gives you more control over these muscles and more sensitivity in the vaginal area—both of which can and often do result in a better sexual experience.

The second effect exercise gives you is stamina and strength, which results in a greater ability to make love longer without getting tired. Third, resistive exercises release stress, making you feel more relaxed and able to give in to your feelings during lovemaking.

Fourth, because these exercises give you the best body you could have, because they make you feel proud of your body, you feel sexier and perhaps less inhibited and more eager to make love.

To understand how these changes in your body affect sexual performance and experience, we go to an expert—Dr. Sandra Aronberg, a gynecologist and obstetrician practicing in Beverly Hills, California, who is an attending physician at Cedars-Sinai Medical Center in Los Angeles and a clinical instructor of obstetrics and gynecology at the University of California, Los Angeles.

According to Dr. Aronberg, it has long been established that muscle control plays a part in sexual intercourse. Back in the 1950s, Dr. Arnold Kegel, who was treating women with bladder-control problems (also called urinary stress incontinence), found that he could avoid surgery to correct this condition by teaching these patients to exercise a muscle in the pelvis called the PC muscle—the pubococcygeus muscle. Without getting too technical, you should know that this is a flexible muscle that forms the bottom of the pelvis and is a sling around the vagina. Dr. Kegel found that not only could women strengthen this pelvic muscle by contraction exercises, but those that did so had an increased capacity for experiencing orgasm. The PC muscle is the actual muscle that contracts back and forth in sexual intercourse, so being able to tighten and strengthen it, to control it, plays a great part in achieving sexual satisfaction and orgasm.

According to Dr. Aronberg, the PC muscle in many women is flabby. As we know from the discussion on muscle use and the need to tone and strengthen muscles to prevent atrophy, the same principle applies to the PC muscle. Exercising this muscle, which plays such a crucial part in sex, is important, easy, and almost always quickly effective.

The exercise in our program called Buttocks and Pelvis (Set I) is perfect for strengthening the PC muscle. It is a simple act of contracting all the muscles in the vaginal area—you release and contract, release and contract, fifty times each morning. If you continue this exercise throughout the day, you improve the chance of quickly toning your PC muscle. It is effective and easy to do, anywhere and any time. Nobody will know you are doing it, and it can easily correct a problem that may be the cause of some sexual dissatisfaction. As a matter of fact, many gynecologists suggest such an exercise to their patients who complain of lack of muscle tone, of feeling too wide inside for their partners and of having an unfulfilling sex life.

If you are not sure of the condition of your PC muscle and are interested in finding out, Dr. Aronberg suggests you speak with your doctor. If you feel uncomfortable talking to your doctor about this, she says that you can try evaluating the muscle yourself by placing two fingers in the vagina and then contracting your muscles in that area. If you feel a contraction on your fingers, that's the PC muscle. If you don't feel anything or only a weak tightening, it could be that your PC muscle needs strengthening.

Another exercise that Dr. Aronberg suggests to increase sexual response is called flicking. Here you contract the same muscles in the vaginal area but you release them quickly. It is similar to the previous exercise except it is done faster, approximating vaginal response during orgasm. A third exercise involves pushing out that whole area, as though you were forcing the vagina out, and sucking it all in. Then repeat. If you have had children, you may remember this exercise from childbirth, but you may not be aware that it is a terrific exercise for tightening all the muscles in the vaginal area.

There are other benefits to exercising the muscles directly involved in sexual intercourse, explains Dr. Aronberg. For example, exercising and contracting the muscles results in increased pelvic vascularity, or blood flow, which in turn causes the vagina area to swell. The more blood that is flowing, the more sensitive the area is to touch. Pelvic vascularity also increases lubrication and seems to increase sexual enjoyment.

By improving the muscle tone, one is also indirectly stimulating the clitoris. It is unusual for the clitoris to come in direct contact with the penis because of the angle the penis enters the vagina. The muscle contraction pulls the clitoris, bringing it down to touch the penis and thus increasing the chance of reaching an orgasm during intercourse. According to Dr. Aronberg, you can improve your sexual responsiveness and your partner's enjoyment by learning to tighten these muscles.

And, as I mentioned earlier, don't dismiss the role that pride in your body plays in a satisfying sexual encounter. If you know the muscles involved in lovemaking are toned, if you are aware of them and can control them (while not necessarily controlling yourself), if you have the confidence, if you know you can sustain sexual intercourse for some time, *and* if you feel sexy and beautiful and proud of the shape and condition of your body, you are maximizing your chances of having a fulfilling lovemaking experience for both yourself and your partner.

EXERCISING FOREVER

Where are you going to move when your body wears out? Putting up a "For Lease: One Body, Used" sign is not practical. Neither is trying to make a trade. What happens when our bodies wear out? If we don't exercise, chances are that the simplest things in the world—like getting up in the morning, playing with the kids, running with the dog, even driving a car—become a strain. It doesn't occur to many of us when we are young that our bodies will not be perfect forever. Not without some help. And if we put off getting into shape, time will eventually run out.

The time to take care of your body is now, no matter how old you are. And once you start, the simplicity of The Body Principal Program will ensure that you keep it up. You can do The Body Principal Program for the rest of your life. You never outgrow it—you don't tire of it, and it never gives up on you. You really can keep your body in great shape. You never have to change the exercise routine—you can, if you want, eliminate or add an exercise, or simply do more of one; you can join in group sports, or take up exercising on machines—but you can keep on doing The Body Principal Program forever. It is a true maintenance program that will give you the best body you can have.

Designed to give you added strength and stamina, to resculpt your body so that it will look the way you want it to, it also works to maintain that wonderful you, no matter how old you are. I am now thirty-three years old. I think I look like a thirty-three-year-old woman—but a thirty-three-year-old woman who is in as good shape as she can be, who works at it every day but who enjoys the exercise and wouldn't give it up for anything in the world. You, too, by maintaining The Body Principal Program, making it a routine and satisfying part of your everyday life, can look and feel your very best, always.

Go for it.